Mohammad Karimi

Spinal cord injury rehabilitation

PAR

Mohammad Karimi

Spinal cord injury rehabilitation

Spinal cord injury rehabilitation based on orthoses, wheelchair, external powered device, functional electrical stimulat

LAP LAMBERT Academic Publishing

Impressum/Imprint (nur für Deutschland/only for Germany)
Bibliografische Information der Deutschen Nationalbibliothek: Die Deutsche Nationalbibliothek verzeichnet diese Publikation in der Deutschen Nationalbibliografie; detaillierte bibliografische Daten sind im Internet über http://dnb.d-nb.de abrufbar.
Alle in diesem Buch genannten Marken und Produktnamen unterliegen warenzeichen-, marken- oder patentrechtlichem Schutz bzw. sind Warenzeichen oder eingetragene Warenzeichen der jeweiligen Inhaber. Die Wiedergabe von Marken, Produktnamen, Gebrauchsnamen, Handelsnamen, Warenbezeichnungen u.s.w. in diesem Werk berechtigt auch ohne besondere Kennzeichnung nicht zu der Annahme, dass solche Namen im Sinne der Warenzeichen- und Markenschutzgesetzgebung als frei zu betrachten wären und daher von jedermann benutzt werden dürften.

Coverbild: www.ingimage.com

Verlag: LAP LAMBERT Academic Publishing GmbH & Co. KG
Heinrich-Böcking-Str. 6-8, 66121 Saarbrücken, Deutschland
Telefon +49 681 3720-310, Telefax +49 681 3720-3109
Email: info@lap-publishing.com

Approved by: Literature of my PhD thesis in Strathclyde University

Herstellung in Deutschland (siehe letzte Seite)
ISBN: 978-3-8473-0583-5

Imprint (only for USA, GB)
Bibliographic information published by the Deutsche Nationalbibliothek: The Deutsche Nationalbibliothek lists this publication in the Deutsche Nationalbibliografie; detailed bibliographic data are available in the Internet at http://dnb.d-nb.de.
Any brand names and product names mentioned in this book are subject to trademark, brand or patent protection and are trademarks or registered trademarks of their respective holders. The use of brand names, product names, common names, trade names, product descriptions etc. even without a particular marking in this works is in no way to be construed to mean that such names may be regarded as unrestricted in respect of trademark and brand protection legislation and could thus be used by anyone.

Cover image: www.ingimage.com

Publisher: LAP LAMBERT Academic Publishing GmbH & Co. KG
Heinrich-Böcking-Str. 6-8, 66121 Saarbrücken, Germany
Phone +49 681 3720-310, Fax +49 681 3720-3109
Email: info@lap-publishing.com

Printed in the U.S.A.
Printed in the U.K. by (see last page)
ISBN: 978-3-8473-0583-5

Table of Contents

2

CHAPTER 1: INTRODUCTION

Spinal Cord Injury (SCI) is damage to the spinal cord that results in loss of mobility and sensation below the level of injury. This disorder is characterized according to the amount of functional loss, sensational loss and of the inability to stand and walk (1-3). The incidence of SCI varies amongst countries. For example there are 12.7 in France and 59 in the United States of America, new cases per million population each year. It may be a result of trauma (especially motor vehicle accident), penetrating injuries, or disease. As a result of this type of disability most SCI individuals rely on a wheelchair for their mobility. They can transport themselves from one place to another using a manual wheelchair with the speed and energy expenditure which is similar to normal subjects (4, 5).

Although, wheelchair use provides mobility to those patients, it is not without problems. The main problems are the restriction to mobility from architectural features in the landscape, and a number of health issues due to prolonged sitting. Decubitus ulcers, osteoporosis, joint deformities, especially hip joint adduction contracture can result from prolonged wheelchair use. SCI individuals often undergo various rehabilitation programmes for walking and exercises. As expected, walking is a good exercise for paraplegics in order to maintain good health; urinary tract infections decrease; cardiovascular and digestive functions improve and psychological health improves.

Several types of orthoses have been designed to enable SCI patients to walk, however they are not without problems which include: independent donning and doffing is difficult, transporting the orthosis from one place to another is difficult, walking speed is reduced compared with 'normal' subjects, cosmesis is poor and the style of walking is abnormal. The speed of walking for a SCI individual using an orthosis is significantly lower than that of an able body person and their energy cost of walking is much higher.

5

Independent and convenient use of the orthosis is important in order that the orthosis be used regularly and successfully. Therefore, functional aspects produced by these orthoses such as ease of standing up and sitting down, donning and doffing the orthosis, ease of access and storage, are important and often leave much to be desired.

Several orthoses have been designed for SCI patients to allow walking as a therapeutic exercise; however the problems of slow walking speed, high energy cost and lack of independent donning and doffing remain serious issues to be resolved. Moreover, the cosmesis of available orthoses is poor and structural stiffness is not sufficiently high to withstand the loads applied on the orthoses without serious structural deformities. Sometimes the mechanical reliability of the orthosis is poor and it is required to be checked regularly. This is a big problem specially for those living far from the rehabilitation centres.

Most SCI patients start walking with orthosis after they received enough treatment to correct the deformities which they have in the knee and hip joints as a result of prolong sitting in a wheelchair. Unfortunately, some patients have knee flexion contracture more than 10 degrees or the knee hyperextension. Since the orthosis can not be used for the patients with more than 10 degrees flexion contracture in the knee joint, some patients have to do special surgical treatment to correct the deformities. This takes lots of time and increases the speed of bone osteoporosis.

One of the orthosis which was designed specifically for these patients is Louisiana State Reciprocal Gait Orthosis (LSU RGO). The original concept of this orthosis was developed by Motloch in 1967 at Ontario Crippled children Centre in Toronto. The original orthosis was made from a couple of KAFOs and a plastic body jacket which were connected to each others by a set of gear mechanism. The mechanical reliability of the orthosis was poor (6). The orthosis was modified and more developed by Douglas in

6

conjunction with Carlton Fillaver Company (FillaverInc USA). The new generation of this orthosis is more cosmetically appending than other available orthoses; however the structural stiffness of the orthosis is not high enough to prevent the deformity and collapse of the orthosis during walking, specially for the heavy patients with high level of spinal cord lesion (7, 8). This problem decreases the efficiency of the orthosis during walking and increases the loads applied on the upper limb trough sticks. Although the functional performance of the subjects in using this orthosis is not as good as other orthoses, many subjects prefer to use this orthosis because of cosmetic reason (7, 9).

Another well designed orthosis which was developed for paraplegic subjects is Hip guidance Orthosis (HGO) designed in Orthopaedic Research and Locomotor Assessment Unit (ORLAU) in Oswestry. This orthosis consists of three main parts, the hip joints, callipers with shoe plates and knee joints, and a body section. The design of the callipers is the same as the traditional KAFO orthosis made of stainless steel with the knee leather straps. According to the results of different research the lateral stiffness of this orthosis is high amongst the available orthoses and it's structural deformity during walking is not too much (8). The functional performance of the HGO orthosis is better in contrast to other well-known orthoses, however many subjects prefer to use other orthoses such as LSU RGO instead. They prefer to use an orthosis which is well fitted on the body and is more cosmetically appending.

Some investigators have tried to design an orthosis which has a structural stiffness the same as that in the HGO orthosis and be as cosmetic as the RGO orthosis. They have tried to use some mechanisms such as using a medial linkage with a couple of KAFOs, using special mechanisms which enable the user to keep both feet parallel to the floor and helping the subjects to move the swing leg forward (Hip and Ankle Linkage orthosis), using hydraulic cylinder to transmit the motion from one side to other side (Hydraulic Reciprocal Gait orthosis), and using air muscles which acts as human muscles to help the swing leg to go forward. In other orthoses such as in Weight Bearing Control orthosis (WBC) a specific control mechanism was used, this mechanism controlled the performance of the orthosis during walking. A motor powered mechanism was attached to the hip joint of the RGO orthosis by Ohta et al (2007) to increase the speed of walking.

The results of different research studies have shown that using the above mentioned orthoses could not improve the ability of the subjects in walking with orthosis. Moreover, they have shown that the HGO orthosis is the best available orthosis for paraplegic subjects. However, many subjects prefer to not use any orthoses or they select other orthoses instead of the HGO, because of cosmetic reason. So designing an orthosis which has a structural stiffness better or the same as the HGO orthosis and be as cosmetic as the RGO orthosis is very important. Designing an orthosis which fulfil these requirements not only improves the performance of the subjects but also, increases their interest to use the orthosis. The new design of orthosis needs to cover the following requirements:

1)   Has a good mechanical reliability

2)   Has a good structural stiffness

3)   The cosmetic of the orthosis be the same as RGO orthosis or better

4)   The weight of the orthosis be less than other available orthoses

5)   Donning and doffing the orthosis be easy for the subjects in order to use the orthosis regularly and independently

6)   Allows the patients with more than 10 degrees of knee flexion contracture to use the device

CHAPTER 2: SPINAL CORD INJURY, INCIDENCE AND FUNCTIONAL SIGNIFICANT

2.1 Introduction

Spinal cord injury (SCI) is damage or trauma to the spinal cord that results in a loss of function, mobility and sensation below the level at which the spinal cord has been injured. This disorder is characterized according to the amount of functional loss, sensation loss and inability of a SCI individual to stand and walk (1, 2).

2.1.1 The annual incidence of SCI

The annual incidence of SCI differs from one country to another; it varies between 12.7 (France) and 59 (USA) new cases per million populations each year (10-15). In Canada, it varies between 37.2 and 46.2 (12). In contrast, it is 40.2, 18, 12.7 and 19.4 new cases per million in Taiwan, Turkey, France and Australia, respectively (10, 13). According to Surkin(13), the incidence of SCI in the USA is 59 new cases per million. However, Wyndaele(15) mentioned that the incidence of SCI in the Northern America is 51. According to the results of the research carried out by Wyndaele, the incidence of this disorder is 19.4 in Europe, 16.8 in Australia, and 23.9 in Asia and 14 in the UK.

In the USA, it is estimated that there are 183,000 to 230,000 individuals living with SCI (16). This prevalence statistics are estimates which was obtained from several studies carried out by different investigators and is not directly derived from National SCI databases. In contrast, the total population of individuals with SCI in the UK is about 40,000. In 1992 there were 900 to 1000 new cases of SCI each year in the UK and it was mentioned that the incidence of this disorder was increasing (11). In Australia the

9

prevalence of SCI varied from 8096 to 9614 cases by 1985. However, by 1997 it was nearly 10,000 people with SCI in Australia (17).

The majority of SCI patients are young, with an age varies between 20 and 40 years (10, 13, 18). Those suffering from SCI in the UK are predominately male (87%) and young (24%, 58% and 72% are teenagers, under 30 and under 40 years old, respectively) (11, 14). In the USA 82% of those patients are male (16). The ratio of male to female with SCI is 5 to 1 in Turkey, however; it is 2.5 to 1 in the rural areas and 5.8 to 1 in Istanbul (18, 19).

2.1.2 The main causes of SCI

The main cause of SCI is trauma, especially road traffic accidents and this is followed by domestic falls, work related accidents and sporting injuries (11, 14). According to O'Connor, motor vehicle collisions were the cause of 50%, falling 37%, work related accident 2%, sports injuries 9% and Iatrogenic 2% of all SCIs in Ireland. He also mentioned in his research that the incidence of this injury is the highest in September followed by May (20).

2.1.3 The types of SCI

There are different kinds of SCI that are named as complete and incomplete according to the types of dysfunction and paraplegia and quadriplegia according to the level of the lesions. According to Maharaj(21) the percentage of complete spinal cord lesion in Fiji is 52% of all cases and nearly 69% of them are paraplegia. In contrast, Karacan stated that nearly 57% of SCI in Turkey have incomplete lesions and 54% of them are paraplegia (18).

10

2.2 The Anatomy of the Spine

The human spinal cord is protected by the bony spinal column, which is made of the bones called vertebrae. These bones are connected together in a way, which allows some motion between them. The vertebral foramina of all vertebrae stacked one in top of the other forms the vertebral canal. This canal is surrounded by parts of the vertebrae and is protected by vertebral ligaments, menisci, and meninge layers (22). The spinal column consists of 33 vertebrae; 7 cervical, 12 thoracic, 5 lumbar, 5 sacral and 4 coccygeal (23). Figure 2.1 shows the anatomy of the vertebral column.

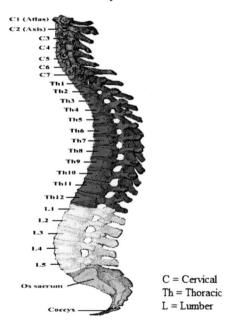

C = Cervical
Th = Thoracic
L = Lumber

Figure 2.1: The structure of vertebral column (adapted from Gray's   anatomy)

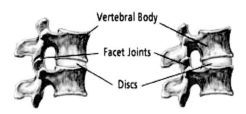

Figure 2.2: The inter-vertebral joints (adapted from Gray's anatomy)

Two strong joints connect each two-adjacent vertebra to each other. The first joint, which locates on the anterior aspect, consists of two adjacent vertebra and inter-vertebral disk. The second joint is on the posterior aspect and is made from pedicle facet joints. The former is actually a weight bearing structure and the later acts as a sliding and gliding joint. Strong ligaments such as the anterior and posterior ligaments, interspinous ligaments and ligamentumflavum support the vertebral column. Some small ligaments such as the dentate ligament also increase the structural stability of the column. Figure 2.2 shows the inter-vertebral joints.

2.2.1 External Anatomy of the Spine

The spinal cord is roughly cylindrical but flattened slightly in its anterior posterior dimension. In infants it extends from the medulla oblongata, the inferior part of the brain, to the third or fourth lumbar vertebra. In the adult, the spinal cord ends at the level of the first lumbar vertebra and hence there is a significant discrepancy between spinal cord segments and vertebral body levels. In the cervical region there is little difference between spinal cord segments and the vertebral bodies and here spinal roots extend from almost laterally out to the inter-vertebral foramens. In contrast, in the thoracic region, the 12 thoracic spinal segments are contained in the upper 9 thoracic vertebrae and the 5 lumbar vertebrae are contained within the canals of T12 and L1 vertebrae. The roots of caudaequina are within the vertebral canal of the lumbar spine. The interesting point is that many muscles of the limbs are predominately supplied by one spinal segment, although two or three spinal segments may also contribute to its innervations. However, some muscles such as pectoralis major, latissimusdoris, serratus anterior and gluteus maximus are real multi segmental muscles. Different spinal segments innervate those, so they may have functionality after an injury of different levels of the spinal cord (22).

2.2.2 Spinal Cord nerves and their plexus

In total, there are 31 spinal nerves, which originate from different levels of the spinal cord and exit through holes named inter-vertebral foramina. The nerves that exit through the spinal column are named according to the level of the foramina from which they emerge. Except for the thoracic nerves from T_2 to T_{12} other ventral rami of spinal nerves combine with each other to make spinal plexuses. There are four spinal plexuses in the vertebral column, which include: Cervical, Brachial, Lumbar and Sacral plexuses.

The cervical plexus consists of the ventral rami of the first to fifth cervical nerves; occasionally a part of the fifth cervical nerve is also in this plexus. It innervates the muscles and skin of the neck and a portion of the head and shoulder. It also has an important role in innervation of the diaphragm, by the phrenic nerve.

The brachial plexus is another spinal plexus, which consists of the anterior rami of the fifth cervical nerve through to the first thoracic nerve, figure 2.3. Some peripheral nerves such as Ulnar, Radial, Median and Musculoskeletal nerves, which innervate upper extremity muscles, originate from this plexus.

13

The lumbar plexus is the spinal plexus which innervates the lower limb muscles. It is formed by the anterior rami of $L_1- L_4$ and sometimes a branch from T_{12}. The nerves which arise from it innervate the structures located in the lower part of the abdomen and the anterior and medial portions of the lower extremity. Many muscles of the lower limbs are innervated by the Femoral and Obturator nerves, which originated from the Lumbar plexus, figure 2.4.

Finally the sacral plexus is formed by the anterior rami of the spinal nerves $L_4- L_5$ and S_1 through S_4. It innervates the lower back, pelvic, perineum, posterior surface of the thigh and leg and dorsal and plantar surfaces of the foot. The sciatic nerve, which is the largest nerve in the body, arises from the sacral plexus. It is composed of the tibial and common peroneal nerves, which innervate some muscles of lower limb, figure 2.5.

2.3 Neurological problems with SCI

Neurological problems occur in the patients with SCI. Distortion of a small portion of the column produces profound motor and sensory change. In complete SCI all function, sensory and motor, is lost below the level of the lesion. In contrast, in incomplete lesions, there is some sensory and motor function below the level of injury.

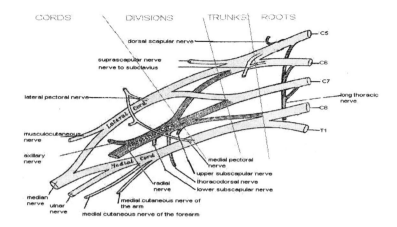

Figure 2.3:Brachial plexus (adopted from Gray's anatomy)

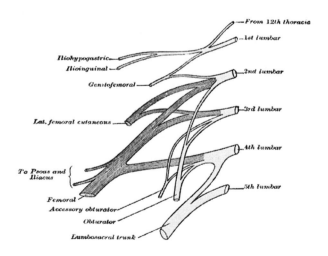

Figure 2.4: Lumbar plexus (adopted from Gray's anatomy)

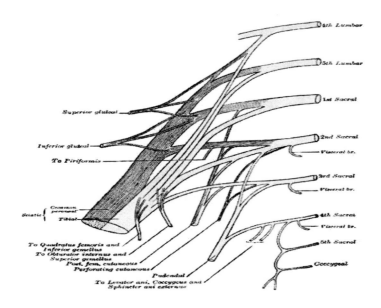

Figure 2.5: Sacral plexus (adopted from Gray's anatomy)

Paraplegia, which refers to any impairment or loss of sensory and motor function in the thoracic, lumbar or sacral segments of the spinal cord, is one of the neurological disorders associated with SCI. It does not affect the functions of the arms; however the function of the trunk, legs and pelvic organs, depending on the level of spinal lesion, may be involved (24-26).

Tetraplegia or quadriplegia is the other neurological disorder, which refers to any impairment and loss of function, sensory and motor, resulting from damage to neural elements within the spinal cord in the cervical region. This happens by any damage to neural elements within spinal cord at that region. As a result, there is loss of function in the arms as well as the trunk, legs and pelvic organs (24-26).

16

There are five specific clinical syndromes that may be associated with incomplete injuries. The first, which is named the Central cord syndrome, is a very common incomplete injury that is associated with greater loss of upper limb function compared to the lower limbs. The second is named the Brown-Sequard syndrome, which results from a hemi section lesion of the spinal cord. This is characterized by relatively greater ipsilateralproprioceptive and functional loss and in the contralateral side there is loss of sensitivity to pain and temperature (24).

Anterior cord syndrome is defined by a variable loss of motor and sensitivity to pain and temperature, with no effect on proprioception. This lesion occurs as a result of any damage to the anterior two thirds of the spinal cord while the posterior part of the column is intact.

Conusmedullaris syndrome results from damage to the sacral cord and lumbar nerve roots within the spinal cord. In this syndrome the sacral reflexes may be preserved. Caudaequina syndrome is as a result of any injuries to the lumbosacral nerve roots, which results in loss of reflexes in bladder, bowl and lower extremities (24).

2.4 Standard classification of SCI

The Frankel system of SCI classification is generally used for SCI description according to the type of impairment (2). The Frankel system is defined as:

 Grade A: complete motor and sensory function disorder
Grade B: motor complete but sensory incomplete function disorder
Grade C: motor and sensory incomplete function disorder
Grade D: useful motor function with or without auxiliary means

Grade E: no motor or sensory function disorder

There is another scale used in grading the degree of impairment of SCI and is actually a modification of the Frankel system. This scale is known as ASIA (American Spinal Injuries Association) system and has one grade for complete injury and three grades for incomplete ones. In this scale the strength of key muscles of the lower limb is used as a factor to determine the grade of injury. Clinicians determine the strength of the muscles by using a five scores scale, in which 0 is applied for total paralysis and 5 for action against a full resistance (24). This system is defined as:

Grade A (complete): is defined as absence of any sensory and motor functions in the sacral segments S4-S5
Grade B (incomplete): sensory is intact but there is no motor function below the neurological level and also sacral segments S4 and S5
Grade C (incomplete): more than half of key muscles below the neurological level have a grade less than 3
Grade D (incomplete): the motor function is intact below the lesion level and half of the key muscles have a muscle score, which is greater or more than 3.

2.5 Functional significance of spinal cord lesion levels

The physical limitations of SCI patients in performing daily activities vary greatly depending upon the level of the lesion. Improvement of some activities such as personal hygiene (bathing, shaving and socially acceptable bowel and bladder function), ambulation transfer (from wheelchair to bed and vice versa), dressing and eating can be achieved by using an effective treatment method (1).

During recent years, different scales have been proposed in order to measure the disability, however the Functional Independence Measurement (FIM) is the most commonly used (3). The ASIA also evaluated this scale in assessment of the functional performance of SCI patients and recommended its universal adaptation in 1994. Table 2.1 shows the parameters selected for FIM as mentioned by ASIA (24).

The first attempt to measure the performance of SCI subjects during daily activities, according to the neurological lesion level was done by Long and Lawton in 1955 and the outcome still serves as a guide today (27).

2.5.1 Functional significance of a spinal cord lesion above the C5 level

Patients with lesion level above C_5 have significant problems with motion and also with breathing. Some muscles such as pectoralis major, latismusDorsi, seratus anterior are inactive in those patients. They have no ability to push their wheelchair and their endurance is significantly low. They are completely dependent on others.

Those with C_1-C_3 lesion level have no movement of the upper and lower extremities muscles. They have only movement of the head and neck or shoulder elevation. They are dependent on others for help with almost all of their mobility and self-care needs. They may be able to use a powered wheelchair with chin or pneumatic controls. It is possible to use different assistive devices which transmit the signals by means of radio waves, infrared waves to control their environment. They may be able to use a powered wheelchair with a Mobile Arm Support (MAS) orthosis to assist them with feeding and grooming activities (1, 24, 27).

Functional Independence Measure (FIM)

LEVELS		No Helper
7 Complete Independence (Timely, Safely)		No Helper
6 Modified Independence (Device)		No Helper
Modified Dependence		
5 Supervision		
4 Minimal Assist (Subject = 75%+)		Helper
3 Moderate Assist (Subject = 50%+)		Helper
Complete Dependence		
2 Maximal Assist (Subject = 25%+)		
1 Total Assist (Subject = 0%+)		

	ADMIT	DISCH
Self Care		
A. Eating	☐	☐
B. Grooming	☐	☐
C. Bathing	☐	☐
D. Dressing-Upper Body	☐	☐
E. Dressing-Lower Body	☐	☐
F. Toileting	☐	☐
Sphincter Control		
G. Bladder Management	☐	☐
H. Bowel Management	☐	☐
Mobility Transfer:		
I. Bed, Chair, Wheelchair	☐	☐
J. Toilet	☐	☐
K. Tub, Shower	☐	☐
Locomotion		
L. Walk/wheelChair	W/C ☐	W/C ☐
M. Stairs	☐	☐
Communication		
N. Comprehension	A/V ☐	A/V ☐
O. Expression	V/N ☐	V/N ☐
Social Cognition		
P. Social Interaction	☐	☐
Q. Problem Solving	☐	☐
R. Memory	☐	☐
Total FIM	☐	☐

NOTE: Leave no blanks; enter 1 if patient not testable due to risk.

ASIA IMPAIRMENT SCALE

☐ **A = Complete:** No motor or sensory function is preserved in the sacral segments S4-S5.

☐ **B = Incomplete:** Sensory but not motor function is preserved below the neurological level and includes the sacral segments S4-S5.

☐ **C = Incomplete:** Motor function is preserved below the neurological level, and more than half of key muscles below the neurological level have a muscle grade less than 3.

☐ **D = Incomplete:** Motor function is preserved below the neurological level, and at least half of key muscles below the neurological level have a muscle grade of 3 or more.

☐ **E = Normal:** motor and sensory function is normal

CLINICAL SYNDROMES

☐ Central Cord
☐ Brown-Sequard
☐ Anterior Cord
☐ Conus Medullaris
☐ Cauda Equina

Table 2.1: Functional Independence Measurement (FIM) adapted from ASIA (24)

SCI subjects with lesion level at C_4 have innervation of the diaphragm, so they may not need use ventilatory assistance. However, those between C_1 - C_3 injuries have to use long term mechanical ventilatory support as a loss of innervation of the diaphragm.

2.5.2 Functional significance of a spinal cord lesion at a level below C_5

Those patients with a lesion level below C_5 have full innervation of trapezius, sternocleidomastoid and upper cervical paraspinal muscles. Some muscles such as those, which rotate and stabilize the neck, are intact in those patients. Rhomboids, deltoids and all of the major muscles of the rotator cuff have partially innervation. These patients have scapular adduction, shoulder abduction, internal and external rotation. The activity of shoulder flexor, extensor and elbow flexor is partially preserved in those patients.

For those with C_5 tetraplegia, a power wheelchair with hand controls can be very helpful for most of their mobility needs. They have problems in using a manual wheelchair, as a result of their reduced respiratory reserved. They need assistance for most self-care, transfer mobility with a manual wheelchair and for socially acceptable bowel and bladder functions (1, 27).

2.5.3 Functional significance of a spinal cord lesion at level C_6

Rotator cuff muscles are fully innervated however; seratus, latissimus and pectoralis major muscles have only partial innervation. Extensor Carpi radialis and flexor Carpi radialis are intact at the wrist. Active grasping is not possible in those patients without using an assistive device. Although the respiratory reserve is low, these patients can move their own wheelchair on a smooth level surface. They need assistance with their

21

daily activities, especially for transferring from bed to the wheelchair and vice versa. They need no assistance for some daily activities such as eating and writing.

2.5.4 Functional significance of a spinal cord lesion at level c_7, c_8

At this level the patient has power in the triceps, common finger extensors, and long finger flexors. Patients with an injury at this level can propel their wheelchair independently on smooth level surfaces. They can transfer from bed to wheelchair and move about in the sitting position. By using an appropriate orthosis to fix the paralysed joints those patients can ambulate to some extent.

2.5.5 Functional significance of a spinal cord lesion at level $T_1 - T_6$

Patients with a lesion at this level have full innervation of all upper limb muscles. Their grip force is good enough to do all their activities in bed independently. They can achieve functional independence of self-care in bladder and bowel function. They need to receive advance training in order to use a wheelchair to move over uneven surfaces. They lack trunk stability and also require help donning and doffing an orthosis. These patients may be able to use an orthosis, such as an HGO, along with a walker and/ or crutches for standing and ambulation.

2.5.6 Functional significance of a spinal cord lesion at level $T_6 - T_{12}$

Patients with a lesion at this level may have strong and powerful upper extremity muscles. The long muscles of the upper back have good innervations and the intercostal muscles are active, so the individuals have good respiratory function and endurance. They can manage bowel and bladder function independently after appropriate training. The patient can use bilateral Knee Ankle Foot Orthoses (KAFO) or HGO orthosis with

22

a walker or crutches for standing and ambulation. They have better trunk control than patients with a higher injury, so they may be able to walk independently with an orthosis. Independent walking requires energy and time; therefore they usually prefer to use a wheelchair for their mobility.

2.5.7 Functional significance of a spinal cord lesion at level T_{12}-L_4

The patients with a spinal cord injury at T_{12} have full innervations of the rectus abdominis, abdominal oblique muscles, transverse abdominis, and all muscles of the thorax. The hip joint hiker (quadratuslumborum) is not active; however some muscles such as the internal and external muscles of the abdomen and latismusDorsi are active for hiking the hip joint during walking with an orthosis. These patients can attempt to walk up and down stairs with orthoses and crutches. Walking with an orthosis places a considerable energy demand on the patient.

For patients with an injury between L_1-L_4, bowel, bladder and ambulation function are impaired initially. With treatment, bowel and bladder function can be independently managed. They can also become functionally independent in terms of household and community ambulation. Orthoses such as ankle foot orthoses and knee ankle foot orthoses can be prescribed for these patients in order to help them to stand and ambulate.

2.5.8 Functional significance of a spinal cord lesion at level L_4-S_2

Patients with a lesion at level L_4 have good muscle function around the knee joint in order to stabilize it during walking. Some muscles such as quadratuslumbarum, lower erector spine and primary hip flexors and quadriceps are intact. However, the major stabilizers of the hip joint are absent and ankles remain frail. The extensors of the knee joint are intact so long leg bracing become unnecessary. The ankle joint is frail and the patients need a suitable AFO orthosis to support it. The lack of hamstring and gluteus maximus muscles increases the incidence of hyperextension of the knee joint in these patients. They can stand and walk using a pair of AFO orthoses. The L_4 patient is completely independent in all phases of self care and ambulation (1, 27).

2.6 Complications associated with SCI

The most common complication of SCI is the loss of functional mobility and sensation below the level of injury. However, paralysis, whether partial or complete, may lead to development of complications in other parts of the body. The following complications can arise in persons with SCI (1):

Respiratory disorder: this occurs as a result of infection in the lungs or from collapse of all or parts of the lungs in SCI subjects. In patients with a lesion at the upper cervical (above C_6) the breathing pattern is altered and patients have difficulty breathing, therefore they need respiratory assistance (1).

Gastrointestinal disorders: gastrointestinal bleeding caused by a stomach ulcer, which relates to stress developed after the SCI.

Cardiovascular disorders: SCI patients have problems related to fluctuating blood pressure. A sudden increase of blood pressure occurs by overdistention of the bowel or bladder and lowered blood pressure occurs when subjects try to stand or ambulate. In these patients, the blood vessels are not able to accommodate the rapid change in posture and cannot maintain adequate blood pressure. Inflammation of the vein followed by formation of blood clots can lead to vascular disease in some individuals (1).

Skin problems: the most common skin problem seen in SCI patients is skin breakdown, commonly known as pressure sores or decubitus ulcers. This occurs as a result of prolonged pressure over bony prominence due to an absence of pain appreciation and an inability of these patients to lift their weight/ posture. The soft tissues over bony prominences such as the greater trochanter, sacrum, knee joint epicondyles and ankle malleoli can be prone to pressure sores (1).

Musculoskeletal problems: the range of motion of the joints decreases if a therapist or other person does not routinely move these joints. Lack of movement can lead to joint contracture, which happens as a result of the joint being in one constant position. Depending on the level of the lesion, the vertebral column may be unstable and a scoliosis may develop.

In normal subjects bone strength is maintained through regular muscle activity and/ or by applying body weight through them. When the muscle activity or when the load applied through the bone decreases, they begin to lose calcium and phosphorus and become weak and brittle. Fractures of long bones secondary to osteoporosis is one of the most common complications associated with SCI (28-30).

Neurological problems: abnormal painful sensation may exist below the level of the lesion. Excessive sweating and spasticity are other neurological problems, which can be seen after SCI (1).

Psychological disorders: some factors such as pain, poor sleep, feeling of helplessness, frequent hospitalisation, poor self-care and problems with transportation increase the risk of psychological disorders (1).

2.7 The benefits of standing and walking for the subjects suffering from SCI

Clinical experience has shown that wheelchair users often have complications secondary to their injury and also due to long term sitting (1). Standing and walking brings some benefits for SCI patients, such as decreasing bone osteoporosis, prevention of pressure sores, and improving the function of the digestive system, which increases their performance during daily activities (31-33).

2.7.1 Decreasing bone osteoporosis

Shortly after SCI, the metabolism changes resulting in the body sending a large amount of calcium and other minerals in the urine. This happens independently of the weight, age and sex of the person. The rate of calcium and mineral loss is high during the first 6-16 months after the injury. Osteoporosis also happens due to the reduction of body weight applied to the bones. Due to spinal cord injury these patients cannot stand and apply load to the lower limb bones, the bones become weaker and thus more brittle. In contrast to the lower limbs, more force may be applied on the upper limbs and spine; as a result the percentage of osteoporosis in the upper limb and spine is significantly less than that in the lower limb bones (29).

In the research carried out by Sabo and his co-workers (28), the Bone Mineral Density (BMD) of the proximal and distal parts of the femur and lumbar spine of 46 male SCI patients, with an average age of 32 years, was monitored regularly. They found a significant difference between the amounts of the BMD of the femur, but not the lumbar spine, between complete and incomplete paraplegic subjects. The level of the BMD of the femur did not show a significant difference between ambulatory and none ambulatory participants. They concluded that the rehabilitation treatment must be for a long time to have a significant impact on the BMD level.

In other research work carried out by Rosenstein (30) the BMD of the upper and lower limbs of 80 myelomeningocel patients, with different levels of lesion was measured. The results of this study showed the effects of the lesion level on the bone density was more in the lower limb than that in the upper limb. They concluded that being ambulatory is an effective factor to decrease bone osteoporosis.

Ogilvie and his co-workers (34) carried out research to evaluate the effects of ambulation with an orthosis on bone density. They followed a group of paraplegic subjects, who walked with an orthosis for a period of 24 months. They found that the BMD of the femoral neck improved or didn't have any change during this period. Standing with an orthosis or in a frame can increase the BMD in lower limb bones and decrease the amount of osteoporosis, which occur in SCI subjects. Although it seems that there is no difference between standing with orthosis or in a frame, the results of the research carried out by Goemaere(35) showed that those who stood with an orthosis had more BMD at the proximal femur in contrast to those who stood in a frame. Fifty three complete traumatic paraplegic subjects participated in this study. The results also showed that the BMD of the paraplegic patients was preserved better in those who stand in contrast to none ambulatory subjects.

It can be concluded that walking and standing increase the BMD of SCI individuals. The effects of standing and walking are more obvious in the lower limb and spine than that in the upper limb. Moreover, standing with orthosis has a better effect on the BMD than standing in a frame. The effect of standing and walking on the BMD is significant if the rehabilitation programmes were followed for a long time.

2.7.2 Prevention of pressure sores

Standing and walking with an orthosis decreases the incidence of skin breakdown in SCI patients (33, 36, 37). The effects of early ambulation with an orthosis on general health were evaluated on 36 patients by Mazur. These patients, who ambulated with the orthosis, had fewer pressure sores and the time of their hospitalisation was less than those using only a wheelchair (37). The subjects, 77% were paraplegic and 23% were quadriplegic, who participated in Dunn et al work (33), also stated that standing in a frame or an orthosis decreased the number of bedsores and improved their independence.

2.7.3 Improvement of respiratory function

It is stated that in the standing position the pelvis tends to tilt more anteriorly than in the sitting position. This increases lumbar lurdosis and establishes a better alignment of the spine in an extended posture. In this posture the force applied on the internal organs decreases and as a result the performance of the respiratory organs increases. During standing, the abdominal organs fall downward and forward, because there is no abdominal muscle function to increase the stability of the abdominal walls anteriorly. As a result the force applied on the diaphragm decreases and respiratory function increases (38, 39). However, the results of the research carried out by Ogilvie (34) showed that orthosis usage and ambulation did not affect the respiratory function of the participants, 24 months after continued use of an orthosis.

28

2.7.4 Prevention of joint deformity

During standing the body weight is applied vertically downward and symmetrically upon both feet. According to Douglas et al (1983), long-term orthosis use and early ambulation after injury decreases the risk of the deformity of the lower limb joints, because it limits the distortions caused by gravitational positioning of the flexed joints. In the work done by Kunkel (40) on a group of SCI subjects, it was found that standing in a frame did not have a significant effect on decreasing muscle spasticity and increasing joint range of motion.

Middleton et al (1997) fitted and trained 25 SCI patients to walk with the 'Walkabout Orthosis' and they were followed up for 2 years. 60% of all participants continued to use the orthosis during their life. Maintained range of motion and prevention of joint deformity were the two most important outcomes, which were mentioned by the researchers (41).

2.7.5 Improving bowel and bladder functions and decreasing urinary tract infections

Decreasing urinary tract infections and improving the function of the bowel and bladder systems are other benefits achieved from orthosis ambulation. In work done by Dunn and his co-workers on a group of paraplegic and quadriplegic subjects (33), they found that standing in a frame or an orthosis, decreased urinary tract infections in the participants and improved their independency to manage sociable bowel and bladder functions.

2.7.6 Improving digestive system function

Another benefit of standing and walking for SCI patients, mentioned in the literature, is the effect on the digestive system function. Eng et al (2001) stated that standing with an orthosis or a frame could regulate and improve the performance of the digestive system. In this research 126 adults with SCI participated. Nearly 30% of them reported that they used their orthoses or frames regularly for prolonged standing, on average 40 minutes per session and for 3 to 4 times per week. They found that standing not only improved the function of the digestive system, but also improved their general health.

2.7.7 Decreasing muscle spasm

Standing with an orthosis or in a frame extends the hip and knee joints and stretches the surrounding muscles. Odeen and Knutsson (1983) showed that standing and applying body weight through the legs reduces muscle spasm more efficiently than stretching the muscles only in the supine position.

2.7.8 Improving independent living

The degree of independence during the performance of daily activities depends on the level of the lesion. The results of the research by Rose et al (1983) showed that the level of independence of SCI subjects improved after standing and ambulation with an orthosis. In an investigation by Syke and his co-workers, the functional performances of 85 patients who were supplied with a Reciprocal Gait Orthosis (RGO) between 1986 and 1993 were evaluated. They found a significant difference between users and nonusers in terms of their assistance needed to do their daily performances (32).

2.7.9 Improving psychological health

Some factors such as poor sleep, problems with transportation, pain and other diseases associated with SCI increase the incidence of psychological health disease (1). Eng and his co-workers showed that the sleep pattern and general health of the participants, 152 adults with SCI, in their research improved with standing (36).

In other work by Kunkel et al (1993), 67% of the participants agreed that standing in a frame had a positive psychological impact on them. Ogilvie in his research mentioned that nearly 33% of the participants were happy with orthosis use and reported a better general health as a consequence of using the orthosis (34).

2.7.10 Improving the function of the cardiovascular system

Improving the function of the cardiovascular system is a further benefit mentioned in the literature concerning ambulation with orthoses; however there is no evidence in the literature to support this view.

2.8 Problems associated with using an orthosis

The main problem with orthosis use is the high-energy demands it places on the user during ambulation. The walking speed of a SCI patient with an orthosis is significantly less than that of normal walking and also in contrast to mobility with a wheelchair. SCI subjects walk more slowly and less efficiently with an orthosis than moving with a wheelchair (4, 42).

It is worth considering that the increased energy consumption during ambulation with an orthosis may have a negative effect on the functional performance of SCI subjects during their participation in social activities. Children with SCI as a result of myelomeningocel could participate in the community or in school activities with a wheelchair but not with an orthosis (43).

CHAPTER 3: ORTHOSIS USED BY PARAPLEGIC INDIVIDUALS FOR STANDING AND WALKING

3.1 Introduction

Different types of orthoses have been designed to enable SCI individuals to walk and stand. The types of orthoses selected by these patients and the type of mechanisms which are used in those orthoses depend on the abilities of the subjects and their level of spinal cord lesion. The following categories of orthoses are used to stabilize paralyzed limbs during standing and walking:

a) Ankle Foot Orthoses (AFO)
b) Knee Ankle Foot Orthoses (KAFO)
c) Hip Knee Ankle Foot Orthoses (HKAFO)
d) Externally powered orthoses
e) Functional Electrical Stimulation (FES)
e) Hybrid orthoses

3.2 Ankle Foot Orthosis (AFO)

Ankle foot orthoses are usually designed to permit safe and effective ambulation of the SCI individuals with lesion levels between L_4 and S_2 (1, 27). They also may be used to prevent the development of deformity and to reduce the effect of spasticity at the ankle joint (44, 45). Using this orthosis during walking may also have significant effects on the knee joint stability (46). The AFOs are divided into two subcategories which include conventional orthoses and plastic orthoses (45, 47).

33

3.2.1 Conventional AFOs

They have a leather covered metal calf band with one or two metal side bars or a posterior bar. The shoe or foot attachment anchors the orthosis distally (44). The distal part of the orthosis is attached into the shoe by means of a stirrup. The ankle joint can have four different configurations such as free motion, dorsiflexion and plantar flexion assist, dorsiflexion and plantar flexion fixed, and dorsiflexion assist ankle joint (plantarflexion fixed). In orthoses used for SCI subjects those with dorsiflexion and plantarflexion fixed and dorsiflexion assist ankle joint are used (45, 48).

A plantar flexion stop at the ankle joint prevents toe drag and stumbling during swing phase however, the ankle angle at which plantar flexion of the ankle joint is locked has a significant effect on the magnitude and duration of the moment applied around the knee joint (45). The flexion moment around the knee joint is greater during walking with the orthosis in which the ankle joint is set at slight dorsiflexion in contrast to orthosis in which the ankle set in a slight plantar flexion angle. However, toe clearance during swing phase of the paralysed foot is improved with an ankle joint which is set in dorsiflexion (45, 49). Figure 3.1 shows the effect of the ankle joint alignment on the amount of the force required to stabilize the knee joint.

Vannini-Rizzoli Stabilizing Orthosis (VRSO) was one of the AFOs designed by the Veterans Affairs Rehabilitation Research and Development Service in 1989, specifically for SCI individuals. It was a new type of below knee orthosis (Boot) which was prescribed for SCI individuals with lesion at T_6 or lower. A full range of motion and stability at all joints of the lower limbs, good function in the upper limbs, good physical abilities with normal pulmonary and cardiovascular status, absence of disease, and having an age of less than 40 were the main criteria for selecting the patients to use this orthosis. The VRSO design immobilized the foot and ankle in approximately 10° to 15°

34

of plantar flexion. The plantar flexion angle of the ankle joint stabilizes the knee joint in extension. There are a lot of contraindications for selections of SCI individuals who can use this orthosis (Kent, 1992). Practically this orthosis cannot be used by most SCI individuals. This orthosis is shown in figure 3.2.

3.2.2 Plastic AFOs

Compared to the conventional types, plastic orthoses are generally more cosmetically appending. They are lighter and offer greater flexibility. The closer fitting and better distribution of pressure are other advantages of this type of orthosis. Variations in ankle movement and degree of resistance to movement depend on the chemical composition and the thickness of the plastic used (44, 47). Plastic AFOs orthoses are made from a variety of thermoplastic and thermosetting materials; such as polypropylene, polyethylene and laminated thermosetting. After introduction of thermoplastic materials, there was a significant decline in the use of thermosetting plastics for orthosis manufacture (45).

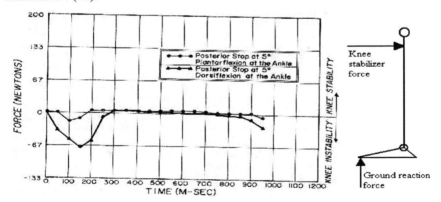

Figure 3.1: The effect of the ankle joint angle on the force required to stabilize the knee joint (45)

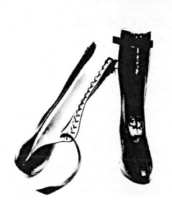

Figure 3.2:Vannini-Rozzoli Stabilizing Orthosis (50)

A rigid AFO is one of the main parts of an RGO orthosis. In order to increase the structural stiffness of the orthosis near the ankle joint, carbon fibre inserts can be used utilizing a vacuum forming technique.

3.3   Knee Ankle Foot Orthosis (KAFO) used by SCI individuals

KAFOs are prescribed for SCI individuals in order that they can stand and walk particularly for those with a lesion level below T_{10} (45). The main purpose of using a KAFO is to stabilize the ankle and knee joints during stance phase. The main components of this type of orthosis include shoes, stirrups, ankle joints and calf band, the same as a traditional AFO, knee joints and thigh section with an anterior soft closure. In the newer designs of KAFOs a plastic AFO is used. Figure 3.3 shows a KAFO which is used by SCI individuals, not seen in the newer version of this book.

36

Different types of knee joints have been designed for KAFOs, such as offset knee joints and knee joints with a ratchet locking mechanism. In the offset knee joint, the axis of rotation is located posterior to the metal uprights. The knee joint is free to move during the swing phase of the gait cycle. This type of knee joint is used for those patients with quadriceps weakness and is not suitable for patients with SCI because they don't have any muscular powers around the knee joints.

The ratchet locking mechanism provides support at limited range of knee flexion, so it is not necessary for the leg to be extended before locking. The ratchet mechanism allows people to stand up in several stages and permits users with knee contractures to be accommodated more easily.

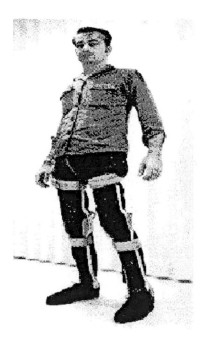

Figure 3.3: Craig-Scott brace design for walking of SCI subjects (44)

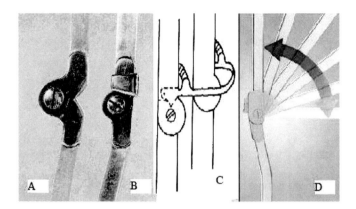

Figure 3.4: Different types of the knee joints, A is an offset knee joint, B is a drop lock, C is a pawl lock knee joint, D is a ratchet knee joint (44)

There is no KAFO orthosis with this type of the knee joint for paraplegics people however, this type of knee joint was used in the Louisiana State University (LSU) RGO orthosis by Solomonow(51). The mechanical reliability of this joint is not high and shearing the teeth occurs as a result of applying excessive force on the gear (48).

The mechanism used to lock and unlock the knee joint also depends on the types of the knee joint. The most commonly used locking system for KAFOs is the drop lock mechanism. The ring drops over the knee joint by gravity or manually by the user, when the mechanical knee is completely extended. Patients who have spasm in the muscles around the knee joint cannot use this locking system. Moreover, sometimes it is difficult to lock the knee joint with this mechanism by the effect of gravity. A pawl lock is another locking system which is easier to release than drop lock, specially when a flexing force is applied on knee joint. A bail which is a semicircular lever placed posterior to the knee joint, unlocks both sides of a knee joint simultaneously by a manual upward pull or by catching the bail on the edge of the chair (44). Figure 3.4 shows different types of knee joints and locking systems.

To maintain full extension of the anatomical knee joint during stance phase some accessory pads and straps are required. The location of those straps is very important to secure the safety of the individual and also to decrease the load applied on the limb during walking. There are six different configurations of straps and bands which can be used for KAFOs orthosis which are:

a) Supra-patellar Strap with Patellar Tendon Strap
b) Lower Thigh Band with Calf Band Closures
c) Lower Thigh Band Closure with Patellar Tendon Strap
d) Supra-patellar Strap
e) Patellar Tendon Strap
f) Knee Cap Strap

Knee ankle foot orthoses can be divided into two main groups: the traditional KAFO and new developed KAFO orthoses. Figure 3.5 shows different types of KAFOs according to the location of the straps.

3.3.1 Traditional KAFO orthoses designed for SCI individuals

One of the best orthosis which was specifically designed for SCI patients was the Craig-Scott orthosis. This orthosis had double uprights, offset knee joints with pawl locks and bail control and thigh and leg bands. The ankle joint of this orthosis had anterior and posterior pin stops. There was a cushion heel in the shoes of this orthosis with specially designed longitudinal and transverse foot plates made of steel (44). Figure 3.3 shows Craig- Scott orthosis.

3.3.2 New KAFO orthosis designed for SCI individuals

The same concept is used in the design of a new orthosis for paraplegic subjects. The main difference between the traditional and the new design of those orthoses relates to the type of materials and knee joint design. One of the new designs of KAFO used for paraplegic subjects was the "New England Regional Spinal Cord Injury Centre" (NERSCIC) KAFO. It was designed by the New England spinal cord injury centre in 1981; it was lighter and more cosmetically appealing in contrast to Craig Scott orthosis. Its AFO component was made from polypropylene by a vacuum forming technique. Figure 3.6 shows this orthosis.

The light weight modular orthosis was another new KAFO orthosis designed for SCI individuals, which was an inexpensive, lightweight, modular orthosis for early standing of patients with paraplegia and quadriplegia. The other advantages of this orthosis were quick fabrication and fitting of the leg frames. It was made from plastic components, AFO and thigh bar, and metal knee joints and assembled with the use of a few tools, straps, and fasteners. The donning and doffing of this orthosis was easier than other traditional KAFO orthoses (52). This orthosis is shown in figure 3.7.

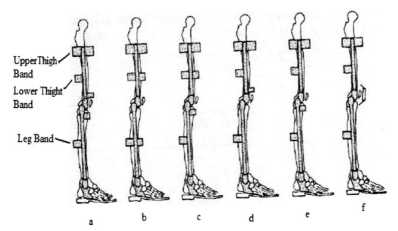

Figure 3.5: Different configurations of the straps that can be used in the Craig Scott KAFO (45)

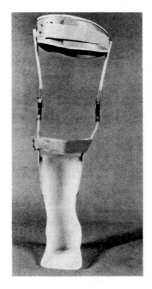

Figure 3.6: NERSCIC KAFO orthosis (53)

41

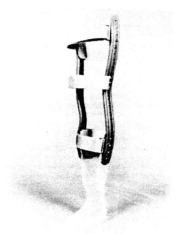

Figure 3.7:The light weightModular KAFO orthosis, suitable for paraplegic subjects (52)

3.4 Hip Knee Ankle Foot Orthosis designed for SCI subjects

Hip Knee Ankle Foot Orthoses (HKAFO) are used to control selected motions of the hip joint using various types of the hip hinges which are inserted between a pelvic band, or a spinal rigid orthosis, and the KAFO (44). The design of these orthoses must provide the following needs (47).

a)   A walking style similar to normal walking
b)   Control of paralysed joints
c)   Increase independency for walking by improving the energy consumption during walking and by decreasing the assistance for sitting down and standing up and donning and doffing the orthosis
d)   Structural integrity

e)   Increasing the efficiency of the users during walking with orthoses with simple walking aids

A variety of mechanical HKAFO orthoses have been designed for paraplegic subjects in order to increase their performance during standing and walking.   The available HKAFO orthoses can be divided into two main groups which are the traditional and the new orthoses.

3.4.1 Traditional HKAFO orthosis designed for SCI individuals

Similarly to other orthoses, the traditional HKAFO orthoses were manufactured from a combination of metal and leather. The hip joint was locked during walking and unlocked for sitting. The most common type of locking system used was the single axis type. Patients walked with this orthosis with a swing through gait pattern. During standing an extended posture of the trunk stabilized the hip joints and decreased the load applied on the crutch. The concepts behind the design of the hip joints for those orthoses were prevention of any motion which the patients cannot control adequately and restriction of the motions which cannot be done in any circumstance during gait cycles, for example adduction and adduction, (44, 47). Figure 3.8 shows the traditional orthosis used for SCI subjects.

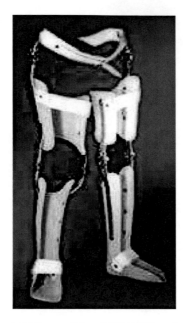

Figure 3.8:The traditional HKAFO orthosis (54)

3.4.2 New HKAFO orthoses designed for SCI individuals

Several new designs of HKAFO have entered into the market since 1971. By employing different mechanisms they allow the SCI patients to ambulate with a reciprocal gait. (48, 55-57).

3.4.2.1Reciprocating Brace with polyplanar Hip Hinges

In all previous orthoses designed for paraplegic subjects, pelvic rotation was not permitted during walking. However, pelvic rotation about the vertical axis is important to increase the step length and to decrease rotation between the foot and the ground. In this orthosis the designer tried to achieve rotation about the vertical axis during walking.

The most practical way to reach to this goal was to displace the axis of the hinge from the horizontal. By using this method in this orthosis, 15 degrees of flexion was combined with 8 degrees of external rotation and 2 degrees of abduction, because the axis of this hinge passed upward and medially. There was another hinge in this system used for sitting, which was aligned along the horizontal axis of the hip joints. However, the polyplanar axis was inserted below the anatomical hip joints with some deviations from horizontal and vertical axis; the hinge axis was aligned at 45 degrees to the horizontal (57, 58).

The stability of the hip joints, mechanical and anatomical, during walking was achieved through using two cable mechanisms. The original concept of this design was from Ontario Crippled Children Centre, Toronto (58). The first cable (A) was attached to the rear of the orthosis side members, so any flexion movement of the legs increased the tension in this cable. By using this cable simultaneous hip joint flexion would be prevented. The second cable (B) was attached to the front of side members of two orthoses so tension in this cable was increased by extension (57, 58). This orthosis is shown in figure 3.9. The main disadvantages of this system according to the designer were as follows:

a) Cable adjustment was necessary every 6_8 weeks
b) With this arrangement of cables and hinges the mechanism was wide

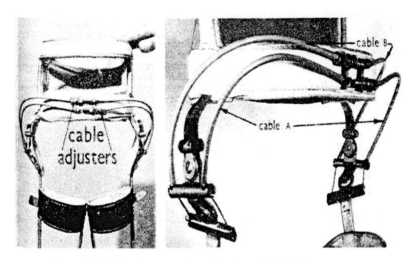

Figure 3.9: Polyplanar reciprocal gait orthosis (58)

This orthosis was tested on the children with myelomeningocel however, it could be used for both adult and child SCI patients.

3.4.2.2Hip Guidance Orthosis (HGO)

A first paper on this topic was presented in 1974 at the inaugural ISPO world congress in Switzerland. This was the first reference to hip joint articulation (59). Major et al (1981) showed the principle of the HGO orthosis which was initially designed for spina bifida children. The design was changed so that the orthosis can be used by adult paraplegics, by using new materials and some improvements in the hip joint (56, 60). After some improvements and changes to the hip joint the name of this orthosis was changed to ORLAU (Orthopaedic Research and Locomotor Assessment Unit) Parawalker. Today both names are used for this orthosis simultaneously.

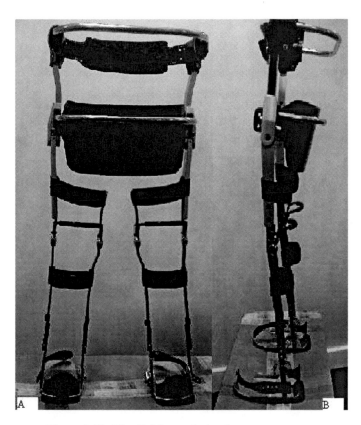

Figure 3.10: Hip Guidance Orthosis

A is the posterior view and B is the lateral view of this orthosis

The HGO orthosis consists of three main parts, which include, the hip joints, callipers with shoe plates and knee joints with pawl lock and bail control and body section. This orthosis is shown in figure 3.10. The specific design of the hip joint in this orthosis, which allows some motion during walking, has the following features (56):

a) It has greater lateral stiffness in contrast to the available orthoses
b) It has less lateral play in walking in contrast to the available orthoses

c) It is easily assembled

d) It is easy to be used by patients

e) It has greater mechanical reliability in contrast to other orthoses

f) It is of lighter weight than other available orthoses

The first design of the hip joint, figure 3.11, was very simple and contained a stop to control the hip joint range of motion in sitting and walking, however it had some problems such as:

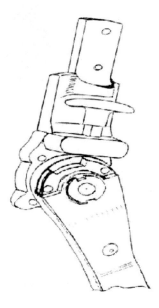

Figure 3.11: The first design of the hip joint used in the HGO (from ORLAU annual report)

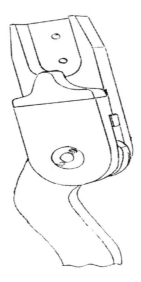

Figure 3.12:The second type of hip joint used in HGO orthosis

a)   The hip joint was cast from aluminium alloy and it was subject to brittle failure

b)   The bearing pin was a cantilever and therefore high bending and shear stresses were applied on it

c)   The formability of the material was not good and it was difficult to shape the lower bar according to the patient's needs

d)   The flexion and extension stops were not adjustable

e)   The maximum range of flexion in the sitting position was 90 degrees

A new hip joint was designed to solve the above problems. It was machined from solid aluminium. In this design an adjustable flexion stop was incorporated and the extension stop was omitted. The range of motion during sitting was increased, by changing the shape of the lower bar of the hip joint. After some changes in this design and incorporating an adjustable extension stop again, the new hip joint was introduced in August 1983, figure 3.12.

The third version of the hip joint was designed in order to improve some features of the previous designs. The mechanical performance of the new design was better than the older ones. It was more cosmetic, easier to manufacture and shape than the older joints. The lower bar of the hip joint had the same shape as the first design. The new more rigid hip joint, figure 3.13, provided an overall increasein lateral stiffness and had a noticeableimproved effect on the walking performance of paraplegic subjects. It was named as the ORLAU Parawalker 89 hip joint. This new design increased the lateral rigidity of the hip joint by 70%. It was shown that increasing the stiffness of the hip joint increased the total rigidity of the orthosis by 10% (61).

The main function of the body brace component is to provide a supporting structure for the leg segment and acts as two of three points of fixation to stabilize the hips. The specific design of this part provides the structural stiffness to the orthosis and improves its rigidity against abduction and adduction moments applied about the hip joint during walking. This component was constructed from two lateral bars with a pair of stainless steel tubes. One tube was bolted to the top of the lateral bars and the other was attached directly to the hip joint, figure 3.13.

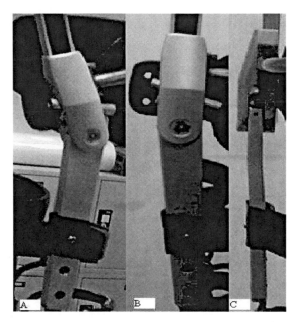

Figure 3.13: The third type of hip joint used for the HGO

A and B are the lateral views and C is the posterior view

The tubes were shaped to the patient's body shape and the body brace was secured to the body by two straps (56). In order to improve the cosmesis and rigidity of the body brace several attempts have been made to manufacture it from composite materials (62, 63).

The KAFOs of HGO orthosis provide the third fixation point for the hip joints. They were manufactured from a machined steel rectangular section. The specific design of the knee joint allows the maximum range of knee flexion in sitting and had a good mechanical reliability. The knee joint of this orthosis had bail lock operation which was easy to use by SCI patients (56).

The shoe plates were attached to the leg segments with approximately 6 degrees of dorsiflexion. It was easy for the patients to don and doff the orthosis and also they could use any shoes they wanted. The security of the ankle was increased by using a polypropylene strap which passed over the mid-foot and fastened via a toggle clamp. The angle between leg segments and shoe plates was fixed and there was no play between them during walking (56).

3.4.2.3 HGO orthosis with composite material body brace

The designers of the Parawalker orthosis paid a lot of attention to increase the structural rigidity of the orthosis in the frontal plane. The main concept behind this was to help the patient to clear the swing leg easily. Due to the greater weight and height of adult paraplegics, the deformation of the orthosis structure is high in this group of patients, so the material which can be used for those patients needs to have enough strength. A crucial factor which influences initial patient choice to select an orthosis is the cosmesis. However, metal body brace is not as cosmesis as to be selected by all patients. To overcome these problems and to decrease the weight of body brace, a new body brace with composite material was developed. The composite material body brace was produced from a mould of the patient, which was taken in an appropriate position and was manufactured by utilizing vacuum forming technique. It was constructed from carbon fibre with aramid fibre to increase structural stiffness of the body segment. It was compared with a metal body brace segment with the same size as the composite one. It was shown that the new design had 40% more lateral stiffness than the metal one. Moreover, it was lighter and was more cosmetically appealing (62, 63).

3.4.2.4 Ortho-Walk Pneumatic Orthosis

This pneumatic orthosis was produced by ILC Dover, a division of ILC industries, figure 3.14. This was a new concept in the field of orthotics however, the mechanism of action was the same as a rigid orthosis. It was used to stabilize the paralyzed joints specially the hip and knee joints during walking. It was a light weight garment that fitted the body snugly. There were two anterior and posterior inflatable tubes which were pressurized to 2.25 kg/cm². It provided enough rigidity to support the body in the upright posture (64). The mediolateral stability and toe pick up during walking was achieved by a plastic AFO orthosis or using special boots (45).

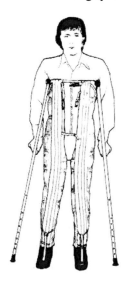

Figure 3.14: Pneumatic orthosis

The pneumatic orthosis was manufactured in 6 sizes and could be easily adjusted for every subject. The weight of this orthosis was significantly lower than a conventional KAFO; the weight of the pneumatic orthosis was 2.27 kg in contrast to the KAFO orthosis which was between 5.45 to 9.07 kg. The walking performance of the SCI

53

individuals during walking with this orthosis could be better if subjects use AFOs as well. It could be used effectively during early mobilization of the SCI since it could be fitted using a suitable size of the patient limbs. This orthosis had some disadvantages such as:

a)   Discomfort of orthosis especially excessive sweating in warm weather and having pain or feeling of pressure in the chest

b)   Inadequate support especially around hip and knee joints

c)   Air leaks and repeated inflation requirement

d)   Zippers: they opened during ambulation

e)   The air pressure was high enough to create pressure sores especially in anesthetic areas

Because of these problems many paraplegics preferred to use other orthoses, especially for higher rates of ambulation (45).

3.4.2.5 Louisiana State University Reciprocal Gait Orthosis (LSU RGO)

The original concept of the reciprocal gait orthosis was developed by Motloch in 1967 at the Ontario Crippled Children's Centre in Toronto, Ontario. He tried to develop an orthosis which could provide stability during standing similar to the Parapodium and also to help the patients in order to walk efficiency. Motloch developed his idea for children with spina bifida. His experimental orthosis was made from a plastic body jacket and a pair of KAFOs which were connected to the body jacket by a set of gears. The orthosis worked, but the mechanical reliability of the gears was inadequate (6).

In a development of this orthosis, Christianson replaced the gear mechanism by double steel cables, which were more durable and effective in contrast to the gear mechanism.

In this generation the hip joints of the orthosis were coupled together using two Bowden cables, so that the extension of one leg produces flexion in other side. In standing, this coupling provides hip joint stability by preventing simultaneous hip flexion. Then Douglas et al (1983) from Louisiana State University developed this orthosis in conjunction with Carlton Fillauer at FillauerInc, Chattanooga Tennessee, to produce the orthosis components commercially. The new generation of the orthosis was developed which was used for patients who suffered from Cerebral Palsy (CP), paraplegia and muscular dystrophy (48, 65). This orthosis is shown in figure 3.15.

Patient selection criteria included those who have: feet without any contractures, knee joints with no deformity of more than 10 degrees and hip joints with no contracture and no limitation for movement. Those patients with contractures in the lower limb joints and with poor upper extremity strength cannot use this orthosis (48).

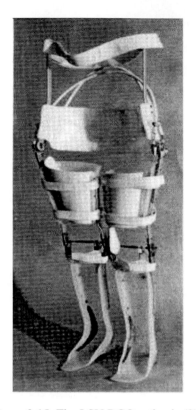

Figure 3.15: The LSU RGO orthosis (8)

The body brace of this orthosis was made of a pelvic band covering the gluteal and sacral areas with two lateral bars and a thoracic extension, which terminated at the xiphoid process. The body brace was secured to the body using two straps. In the new design a custom moulded plastic girdle is used instead of a traditional pelvic band. It helps to distribute the pressure over a greater area and has superior sitting comfort (48).

In the first design, the knee joints were of posterior offset type with ring locks on their lateral sides. In the new design other types of knee joints such as swivel knee joints were used. In the orthosis which is designed for children the medial knee joint may be omitted and a drop lock knee joint used for the lateral side. The posterior thigh shell was manufactured from polypropylene, which was formed over plaster models of the patient's legs. The AFOs of this orthosis were made from polypropylene and were reinforced in the ankle area with composite inserts (carbon fibre) to assure stability against dorsiflcxion. The ankles were placed in the plantigrade position in this orthosis. The Velcro knee control strap was fitted at mid patellar tendon level in order to maintain the knee joint in an extended position (48). The components of the RGO orthosis are produced commercially by FillauerInc, USA.

3.4.2.6Steeper Advanced Reciprocal gait Orthosis (ARGO)

The ARGO orthosis, figure 3.16, was developed by Hugh Steeper Ltd, London, UK and was actually a modified LSU RGO orthosis. In this orthosis only one posterior cable was used and also the hip and knee joints in the same side were connected to each other. This orthosis is commercially available and consists of two moulded polypropylene AFOs with lateral uprights. Those lateral uprights extend from the AFO through the hip joints to chest height. The body brace consists of two lateral bars with a rigid cross bar at the distal end. Jefferson and Whittle (1990) established that the inclusion of a compression mechanism in the ARGO orthosis made sitting and standing easier than other available orthoses. It has benefits to the patients both socially and in terms of energy expenditure at the beginning and ending of walking .The method of walking in the ARGO is the same as that used in the LSU RGO orthosis (8).

3.4.2.7Adjustable ARGO orthosis

This orthosis, based on the ARGO orthosis, was designed by Scivoletto et al (2003) in the Catholic University, Italy. The difference between the ARGO orthosis and this orthosis were that the height; distance between ground and hip hinge, and width, the distance between the hip joints of the orthosis, were adjustable according to the size of the patients (66). Figure 3.17 shows this orthosis. This orthosis is no longer in use.

3.4.2.8ARGO Orthosis aligned in a slight abduction

The concept of an orthosis which is aligned in abduction to decrease the amount of the lateral sway of the body during walking was investigated by Stallard and Major (1993). It was also expected that alignment of the orthosis in a slight abduction decreased the amount of force required to stabilize the stance leg and also yield better utilization of the swing crutch force for propulsion. Some researchers used some mathematical descriptions of the mechanical stress at the hip hinge to determine the best mechanical abduction angle which can be used in the hip hinge of the orthosis (67). Rose was cited by Ijzerman that the best abduction angle for an orthosis is 5 degrees; however the author is of the opinion that an optimal abduction angle must be determined for each subject individually. In this orthosis, which was based on ARGO orthosis, the angle of abduction differed from 0 to 9 degrees and this was achieved by using different 'bent rods' aligned in abduction of 0, 3, 9 degrees (67). Those bent rod are shown in figure 3.18.

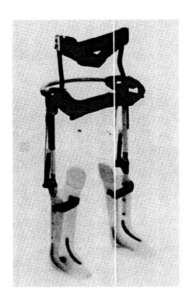

Figure 3.16: ARGO orthosis suitable for walking of paraplegic subjects (8)

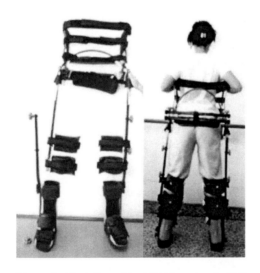

Figure 3.17: Adjustable ARGO orthosis (66)

3.4.2.9 Isocentric Reciprocal Gait Orthosis (IRGO)

The IRGO was also a modification of the LSU RGO. In this orthosis, the two crossed Bowden cables were replaced by a centrally pivoting bar and tie rod arrangement. The rigidity of this orthosis was greater than the LSU RGO orthosis and the friction of system was less than that of the LSU RGO. Davidson (1994) showed that friction in the IRGO was between 2 and 3 times less than that in LSU RGO orthosis, so it was shown that the performance of the subjects with this orthosis could be better than with RGO (68). This orthosis is shown in figure 3.19.

3.4.2.10 Four- Bar Gait Control Linkage Orthosis

This orthosis was designed by David and Rolfes (1981) for a patient who had spastic paraplegia with modified Brown –Sequard syndrome at level T_3. The patient was unable to control severe hip adduction in the upright position with bilateral knee ankle foot orthoses. This problem was solved by using a device which was called as the four bar gait control linkage. The scissor deformity during walking was solved and the patient could walk with a reciprocal gait pattern. The linkage was made from two aluminium and two steel bars with three thrust bearing joints. The middle joint was inserted three inches above the knee joint and attached via the stainless steel bars to the medial upper upright of the KAFO orthosis. By using this orthosis, the patients could walk independently and with a reciprocal gait pattern (69). Figure 3.20 shows this orthosis.

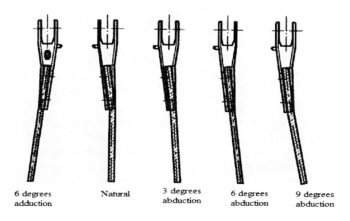

| 6 degrees adduction | Natural | 3 degrees abduction | 6 degrees abduction | 9 degrees abduction |

Figure 3.18:The bent rods used for the ARGO (67)

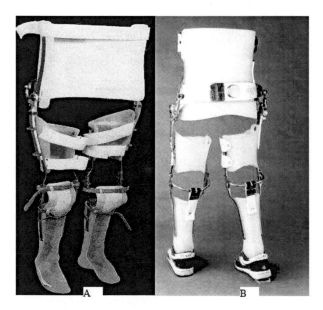

Figure 3.19: The IRGO for SCI subjects, A is anterior view and B is posterior view (68)

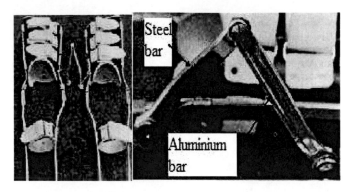

Figure 3.20: Four bar linkage orthosis (69)

3.4.2.11 Medial linkage orthosis (MLO)

This orthosis was designed by McKay and was named the 'Walkabout Unit'. It consisted of bilateral KAFO orthoses with a medial single axis hip joint. Specifically this unit prevented adduction of the swing leg while the body was tilted to clear the swing leg from the ground and also stabilized the supporting leg under the body weight. The 'Walkabout Unit', it refers to the hinge, was placed below the perineum and was not aligned congruently with the centre of the hip joints. There was a discrepancy between the mechanical hip joint axis and anatomical one between 100 mm and 150 mm in this orthosis (70, 71). The relative motions between the orthosis and the body of the subject decrease the performance of the orthosis during walking. It seems that the huge discrepancy between the centre of the motion of the mechanical and anatomical hip joints decreases the stride length during walking.

The KAFOs were manufactured individually and were made similar to other standard commercially available KAFOs. This orthosis has some advantages such as being light weight, easy to don and doff and easy to be used with a wheelchair. The short stride length and horizontal rotation of the pelvis in walking were the two main disadvantages of this orthosis (72). This orthosis is shown in figure 3.21.

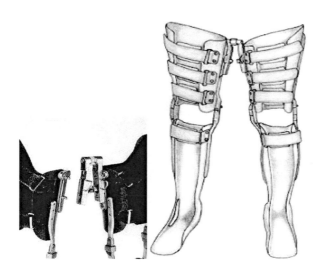

Figure 3.21:The Medial Linkage Orthosis used for SCI subject walking (71)

3.4.2.12Moorong Medial Linkage Orthosis (MMLO)

This orthosis was designed with the same concept as the MLO. Whilst attempting to compensate further discrepancy between the mechanical hip joint and anatomical one in the MLO orthosis, Kirtley pointed out that "due to the length of the limb which is nearly one metre and the range of motion of the hip joint in this system, which is limited, only a small amount of soft tissue distortion is required to accommodate the discrepancy between both mechanical and anatomical hip joints" (70). However, this amount of discrepancy increases the resistance against leg motion and decreases the hip joint range of motion during walking with this orthosis. In this new orthosis (MMLO) the distance between the hip joint centre and the hinge axis of the MLO was decreased by using a curved sliding link centred on the hip joints. The hip joint axis in this orthosis moves along a circle that coincides better with the anatomical hip joint (70). This orthosis is shown in figure 3.22.

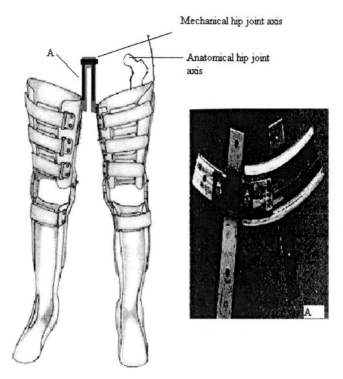

Figure 3.22:Moorong MLO orthosis (left side) and hinge used in this orthosis (A) (70)

3.4.2.13Hip and Ankle Linkage Orthosis (HALO)

A further problem of the MLO according to Genda et al (2004) may be related to lack of a mechanism to assist hip joint flexion and the ankle joints which have no motion during walking. These problems increase the instability especially when the step length becomes longer. This problem was solved by using a mechanism that enables the user to keep both feet parallel to the floor and assists the swinging of the leg by dorsiflexion of the ankle on the stance side.

The new orthosis was named as Hip and Ankle Linkage Orthosis (HALO) and consists of a medial single axis hip joint and two KAFOs. The hip joints had two pulleys with the same axis, however they worked independently. The pulley of the left side was connected to the KAFO of the right side and the pulley of the right side was connected to the KAFO of the left side. In this orthosis the heels of both sides were connected to the hip joints by steel wires. A wire from the left heel was attached to the left hip pulley (right KAFO) and another wire attached the right heel to the right pulley (left KAFO). There was another wire in this system which linked the forefoot sections of both AFOs. As a result plantarflexion of both feet at the same time was impossible. (72). Figure 3.23 shows this orthosis.

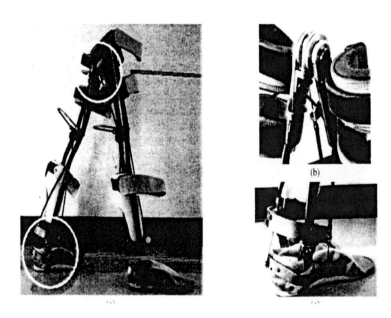

Figure 3.23: HALO orthosis (72)

3.5 Hydraulic, pneumatic and electrical powered orthosis designed for SCI individual

Different types of orthoses have been designed for the SCI subjects which used hydraulic or pneumatic control systems or electrical sources of power to help the patients to move their limbs forward during swing phase. Many of those orthoses were only evaluated in the laboratory and have not been produced commercially. Those orthoses include:

a) Hydraulic Reciprocating Gait Hip Knee Ankle Foot Orthosis (HRGO) designed by Ozyalcin and Ozbasli (1992)

b) Pneumatic Active Gait Orthosis (PAGO) designed by Belforte et al (2001)

c) Powered Gait Orthosis (PGO) designed by Ryu et al (2004)

d) Weight Bearing Control Orthosis (WBC) designed by Yano et al (1997)

e) Two degree of freedom motor powered gait orthosis designed by Ohta et al (2007)

f) Driven Gait Orthosis (DGO) designed by Hocoma

3.6 Functional Electrical Stimulation

Functional Electrical Stimulation (FES) is the application of external stimulation to paralysed muscles to restore their function. Patients with an injured central nervous system often have total or partial paralysis of their extremities; however they have an intact peripheral neuromuscular system. Many attempts have been made to restore the loss of functions by stimulation of the peripheral neuromuscular system artificially. There are three different types of stimulation which include:

a) Electrical stimulation of ventral roots

b) Electrical stimulation of peripheral nerve

c) Electrical stimulation of the muscles themselves

The stimulation electrodes may be applied on the skin, through the skin and also they may be implanted. Transcutaneous stimulation, using electrodes on the skin, is the easiest method to apply. It is used predominantly for stimulation of the common peroneal nerve in patients with drop foot. The main difficulty with stimulation is that the muscle force decreases after several stimulations.

In percutaneous stimulation, thin coiled wires are inserted through the skin into the muscles. This is done via a hypodermic needle. The main advantage of this type of stimulation is that unique muscles can be selected. However, electrode leads may break and care should be taken to prevent infection of the skin at the site of leads. The implanted electrodes may be used for direct muscles stimulation or nerve stimulation. The advantage of nerve stimulation is the possibility to stimulate several muscles from one position. However, the main problem with this type of stimulation is that sometimes the balance between different groups of muscles innervated by a nerve fibre is disturbed. Inefficient muscle contraction, fast muscle fatigue and poor control of muscle force are other disadvantages of this method of stimulation (73).

3.7 Hybrid orthosis

The hybrid orthosis is a combination of a mechanical orthosis such as the ARGO, HGO, LSU RGO, and IRGO with a Functional electrical stimulation (FES) system. Researchers have planned to combine mechanical orthoses with FES to provide prolonged standing and ambulation with minimal energy consumption and applied loads on the upper limbs (61). FES standing and walking are restricted because of inadequate power produced by stimulated muscles. Mechanical orthoses are used with FES systems to control and stabilize frail joints (hip and knee joints) and to reduce the fatigue of the muscles during walking (74, 75). Four different applications of FES may be used in these orthoses which include:

a) Reciprocal electrical stimulation of quadriceps and hamstrings muscles

b) Electrical stimulation of the gluteus and hamstring muscles, on the stance side

c) Electrical stimulation of gluteus muscles on the stance side

d) Electrical stimulation of quadriceps femoris, gluteus maximus, gluteus medius, tensor fascia latae, iliopsoas, sartorius and gracilis.

Theses hybrid orthoses are divided into two main groups according to the types of the orthoses which include: available orthoses and new designed orthoses.

3.7.1 Hybrid orthosis based on the available orthoses

Butler and Major (1987) were the first researchers who used FES system with an HGO orthosis. They tried to increase the structural stability of the orthosis during stance phase by stimulation of paralyzed gluteal muscles to provide abduction and extension moments around the hip joints during walking. A simple stimulated mechanism was used, which was operated by patients by using switches attached to the handle of the crutch. The results of this research showed that although the Force Time Integral (FTI) of the crutch force decreased by between 25 and 50 % in contrast to walking with the HGO, it had some problems associated with FES which include:

a) The contraction of abdominal wall muscle associated with gluteus muscles stimulation

b) Difficulty in connecting electrodes accurately

c) Inconvenience of the cable connecting the control switch on the crutch to the stimulators

Using FES with the HGO orthosis was not successful and participants preferred to use the mechanical orthosis without electrical stimulation (76).

FES system was also used with the RGO, IRGO, and MLO orthoses in order to increase the performance of the paraplegic subjects during walking (77-80). Ferguson et al (1999) showed that walking with a hybrid orthosis based on IRGO was perceived to be significantly easier and faster than walking with the orthosis without stimulation. In contrast Sykes et al (1996) mentioned that using FES with RGO orthosis did not increase RGO use and it did not increase the performance of the subjects in walking with the orthosis.

In summary, the performance of the subjects in walking with hybrid system based on the available orthoses is not significantly improved in contrast to that with the mechanical ones. Moreover, using stimulation has some disadvantages such as difficulty in connecting electrodes accurately, muscle fatigue, and inconvenience of the cable connection.

3.7.2 Hybrid orthosis based on the new orthoses

A variety of new orthoses have been designed which specifically focused on producing the knee motion during swing phase and locking it during stance phase and, also in controlling the motion of the hip joint during walking. The main difference between the new designed orthoses is related to system which was used to control the motion in the hip and knee joints. The new designed hybrid orthosis include:

a)   Modular hybrid orthosis designed by Andrew (1990)

b)   Spring Brake Orthosis (SBO) (81)

c)   Hybrid orthosis with new knee and ankle joints flexion component (82)

69

d)   Wrapped Spring Clutch Orthosis (WSO)(83)

e)   Hybrid orthosis designed by Baardman et al (2002a, 2002b)

CHAPTER 4: GAIT ANALYSIS OF ABLE-BODIED

4.1 Introduction

Walking is one of the most important forms of human locomotion. Gait analysis is the term applied to measuring, analysis and assessment of the biomechanical parameters and events which happen during walking. The study of different aspects of gait analysis started from the times of Leonardo da Vinci (1452-1519), Galileo (1564-1642) and Newton (1643-1727). The movement of the Centre of Gravity (COG) and the mechanism of balance during walking were described scientifically by Borelli in 1682. The first clear description of the gait cycle was produced by the Weber brothers in 1836 in Germany. Newton, Galileo and others had good descriptions of the events which happen during walking. Further progress followed by the development of the force platform which has contributed greatly to the scientific study of gait. It measures the direction and magnitude of the ground reaction force beneath the foot (84, 85).

Walking requires antigravity muscular support, joint mobility to allow smooth progression, and adequate motor control for the transition of body weight from one limb to the other. Disturbance of normal walking may be caused by disease, trauma, degeneration, fatigue, or pain, which restricts normal activities.

4.2 Terminology used in gait analysis

The gait cycle is defined as the time interval between two successive occurrences of one event of walking. The commonly chosen repetitive event in the gait cycle is heel contact of one foot, especially the right foot. The gait cycle is divided into two major parts, which are named as stance, when the foot is in contact with the ground, and swing,

71

when the foot is moving forward through the air. The major subdivisions of the stance phase include:

a)   Heel contact (first double limb support)
b)   Mid stance (single limb support)
c)   Terminal stance (second double limb support)

The swing phase is subdivided into the following parts:

a)   Initial swing
b)   Mid swing
c)   Terminal swing

The stance phase, which is also named the support phase, lasts from heel contact to toe off. Heel contact of the right foot occurs when the left foot is still on the ground. This is actually the first double limb support phase, which is followed by a plantarflexion of the ankle joint to get the entire foot on the ground. The next stage is mid stance in which the body weight is applied completely through the foot in contact with the ground and is a period of the single limb support. In terminal stance the heel leaves the ground and the ankle begins to propel the body forward.

The swing phase, which is between 38 and 40% of the gait cycle, starts with initial swing. In initial swing the lower limb moves forward with a positive acceleration and then followed with mid swing in which the leg is under the body, beside the stance foot (86). Finally in terminal swing the acceleration decreases and the foot reaches to a position to start the next heel strike. Figure 4.1 shows the different subdivisions of the gait cycle.

The stance phase lasts 60% to 62% of the gait cycle (85, 86). In stance phase each double limb support is considered to be 10% of the total gait cycle and 40% of the cycle is single limb support, which is nearly equal to the swing of the other leg however, when the speed of walking increases the time of double support decreases. The terms used to describe the placement of the foot on the ground include:

Stride length: is the distance between two successive placements of the same foot

Step length: is the distance between two successive placement of right and left foot, for instance the distance between heel contact of the left foot and heel contact of the right foot.

Walking base: is the side to side distance between the lines of the two feet. It is measured usually at the midpoint of the heel however; it can also be measured below the centre of the ankle joint.

Toe out: is the angle between the reference line, which is the line between the second toe and the middle point of the heel, and the line of progression during walking.

There are other terms used to describe the linear measurement of the gait cycle, which include:

Cadence: is the number of steps taken in a given time (minute).

Walking speed: is the distance covered by the whole body in a given time. It is measured in metres per second or metres per minute.

An extensive study of gait maturation was carried out by various researchers. The results of those studies showed that gait parameters such as cadence, stride length, walking speed and range of motion of different joints are age dependant. In the work done by Murray and her co-workers (87) the gait parameters of 60 subjects with different ages were analysed repeatedly. They found a significant difference between the mean values of the gait parameters between different age groups. Table 4.1 shows some results of this work. In another study by Kadaba(88) the kinematic parameters of the lower extremity during level walking was measured for 40 female and male participants. The results of this study showed that although the cadence of females was more than that of males, they walked slower than males. The stride length of the women was shorter than that of the men. The percentage of double limb support was the same between men and women in that research, table 4.2. The stride length of the participants in Murray's work differed between 1.53 and 1.588 metre however, it varied from 1.3 to 1.41 metre in the research of Kadaba. The walking speed of the participants in Murray's work was more than that in the research carried out by Kadaba et al.

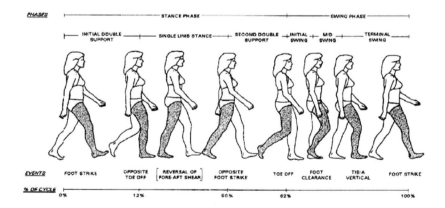

Figure 4.1: Typical normal walking cycle and its subdivisions (84)

74

Age groups	Numbers of observations	Swing phase %	Stance phase %	Double support %	Stride length (cm)	Cadence (steps/min)	Walking speed (cm/s)
20-25	48	40	60	9	158.8	115	153
30-35	48	39	61	11	156.9	111	145
40-45	48	39	61	11	155.9	122	159
50-55	48	40	60	10	157.9	118	155
60-65	48	39	61	11	153	115	147

Table 4.1: : The gait parameters of healthy men who participated in study by Murray (87, 89)

parameters	Cadence (steps/min)	Velocity (m/s)	Stride length (m)	Stride time (second)	Stance phase %	Double limb %
Males	112± 9	1.34± 0.22	1.41± 0.14	1.08± 0.08	61± 2.1	10.2 ± 1.5
Females	115± 9	1.27± 0.16	1.3± 0.1	1.05± 0.08	60.7 ± 2.6	10 ± 1.4

Table 4.2: The gait parameters of 40 healthy men and women measured by Kadaba(88)

In the research carried out by Murray only male participants were selected however, in the research by Kadaba two groups of men and women were selected. The main reason for the difference between the stride length and other Spatio-temporal gait parameters between those stated in their research was related to the participant sexuality. As was shown by Kadaba et al the gait parameters of the females differ from males'.

4.3   Joint motion during level walking

During gait important movements occur in different joints in all three planes, sagittal, frontal and transverse. Each part of the limb has a specific pattern of motion which it follows repeatedly during walking. For example, the upper body moves forwards

75

throughout the gait cycle. The shoulder girdle has a twisting motion which is in an opposite direction to that of the pelvis during normal walking. The trunk also has a side to side motion, once in each cycle in order to increase the stability of the leg during walking. The motion of the pelvis differs from that of shoulder girdle; it twists around the vertical axis and also displays forward and backward tipping which is in associated with a change in lumbar lordosis. The motions of the pelvis during walking can be seen in figures 4.2, 4.3 and 4.4.

Maximum hip flexion occurs between the middle and end of swing phase (85). At the beginning of the stance phase it is in 30 degrees of flexion and then after weight bearing it starts to extend and reach its maximum extension at appropriate contralateral foot strike, then starts to flex in order to transfer body weight to the other limb. In the coronal plane it is in a neutral position (not in abducted or adducted position) at foot strike and then it adducts rapidly however, it returns to an abducted position at the end of stance phase. In swing phase, the hip joint starts to adduct and reaches to the neutral position at the end of the gait cycle. The motion of the hip joint in sagittal and coronal planes can be seen in figures 4.2, 4.3, and 4.4.

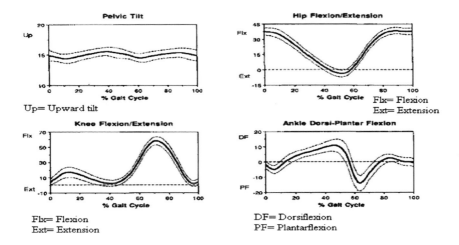

Figure 4.2: The motion of the pelvis, hip, knee and ankle joints in the sagittal plane,

men with different age groups, according to the research by Kadaba(88)

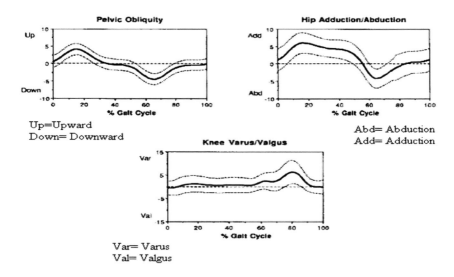

Figure 4.3: The motion of pelvis, hip and knee joints in the coronal plane during level

walking, according to the research by Kadaba(88)

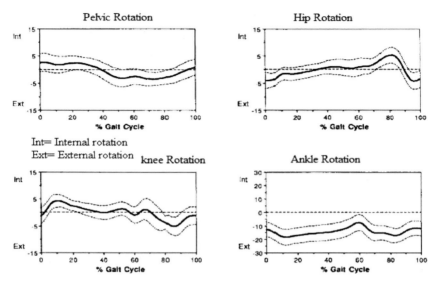

Int= Internal rotation
Ext= External rotation

Figure 4.4: The motion pattern of the lower extremity in transverse plane   during
level walking (88)

In swing phase, the hip joint changes its rotational direction from internal rotation into
external rotation, however in the stance phase it is in an externally rotated position and
reaches its neutral position in terminal stance. Figure 4.4 shows the rotational motion of
the hip joint during walking.

The knee joint has two flexion and two extension patterns in each gait cycle. It is in an
extended position before heel contact, it then flexes early in the stance phase, as soon as
the body weight is applied on the leg. It goes to extension in mid stance and then flexes
at the end of stance phase and reaches its flexion peak during initial swing (84, 85, 88).
The motion of the knee joint, in the sagittal plane, during normal walking can be seen in
figure 4.2.

78

The knee joint has both abduction and adduction motion within each gait cycle. During stance phase it is in neutral position, not in abduction or adduction position, although it has a little abduction, as soon as body weight is applied on the limb. In swing phase the knee joint starts to adduct however, it reaches to a more neutral posture at the end of the swing phase. The pattern of motion of the knee joint in the transverse plane is nearly the same as that for hip joint. It starts to rotate internally at the beginning of the stance phase and reach to its peak before mid-stance. Then it rotates externally up to the terminal stance and rotates internally at the beginning of the swing phase and finally has an external rotation in the swing phase (84). The pattern of motion of the knee joint in the coronal and transverse planes during level walking can be seen in figures 4.3 and 4.4.

The ankle joint is almost in the neutral position, when foot strike occurs, it then plantarflexes, as body weight is applied on the limb. In mid stance the ankle is in dorsi flexion, and in the terminal stance it reaches to plantarflexion again to transfer body weight to the contralateral leg. During swing phase, the ankle joint is in a dorsiflexed position to decrease the length of the limb and to prevent contact of the swing foot with the ground (84, 85, 88) . Figure 4.2 shows the motion of the ankle joint in sagittal plane during normal walking.

The other motions of the ankle joint complex in transverse and frontal planes depend on the foot motion. It is in an external rotated position during stance phase however, it rotates slightly inward when the body weight is transferred upon the other leg. During swing phase it remains in an externally rotated position (88). Figure 4.4 shows the motion of ankle joint during walking in the transverse plane.

4.4   Ground reaction force during walking

Ground reaction forces are actually responses to the force which are produced by muscles and the weight of the body transmitted through the foot. Those forces, which can be measured by using a force plate, are represented as three components, which are:

F_x = Anteroposterior component

F_y = Vertical component

F_z = Mediolateral component

The vertical component of the ground reaction force (GRF) is equal to the force of the body's weight plus the force of acceleration of the Centre of Gravity (COG). When the COG accelerates downward, the vertical component is less than body weight however, during upward acceleration it is more than that of body weight. The first maximum peak in the vertical GRF in the typical plot of this force occurs during the first double stance phase and it is nearly 120% of body weight. During single limb support the vertical component of GRF decreases to about 80% of body weight. There is another peak in the vertical component which occurs at the second double limb support (84, 86).

The anterior-posterior (AP) force is first a braking force and then a propulsive force. The maximum magnitude of this force is approximately 20% of body weight. The area below this curve is the impulse of the force. The braking impulse and propulsive impulse should be approximately equal for symmetrical gait.

The maximum value of the mediolateral GRF is usually 5% of body weight, which is significantly less than that of the AP force. It should be mentioned that this force is in a medial direction in the first part of stance phase and then in a lateral direction in the second part of this phase (86, 90). Figure 4.5 show the force applied on the foot during normal walking.

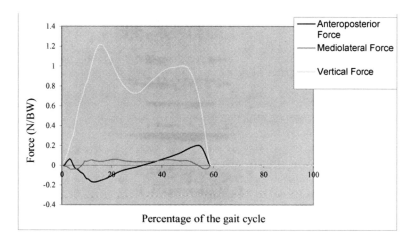

Figure4.5: The Ground reaction force applied on the foot during normal walking

CHAPTER 5: GAIT ANALYSIS OF SPINAL CORD INJURY SUBJECT

5.1 Introduction

The gait mechanism selected by spinal cord injury subjects, depends on the level of their lesion, type of lesion and their ability to walk. However, the most common ones are four –points, swing through gait, swing to gait, reciprocal gait and drag-to patterns. There are three mandatory components for locomotion (47). These include:

a)   Stabilization of multi segmental structure, it can be done intrinsically or extrinsically

b)   Propulsion power. This can be supplied by muscular contraction or by using external power sources

c)   A system to control both a and b

The stability of a multi segmental structure like the human body is achieved by using muscles in the normal and by using orthoses and crutches in handicapped subjects. Depending on the orthosis, different mechanisms are used to increase the stability during standing and walking. They can be done by stabilizing the paralysed joints, such as the knee and ankle joints in Knee Ankle Foot Orthoses (KAFO) or by restricting the range of motion, which is used in the hip joints of the RGO and HGO orthoses. In some orthoses such as the HGO the structural stiffness of the orthosis guaranties the mediolateral stability of the hip joints during standing.

The source of power during normal walking is muscular force which is injected to the hip joint during first part of the stance phase however, in paralysed subjects it is enhanced by using pneumatic, hydraulic or electrical powers. In the other orthosis such

82

as the HGO the force of the upper limb muscles is transmitted to contralateral hip joint to move the hip joint into extension (60).

In order for stability and propulsion to be maintained, a control system is required to maintain the pattern of energy production and the amount of body stability. Feedback from the sensory or non-sensory interface is one of the important control systems which is used during normal walking and walking of a paraplegic subject with an orthosis. Some structural parameters, such as hip joint articulation with a limited range of motion or by using a cable are extrinsic control systems selected by the orthotic designer in order to improve the function of the orthosis (48, 55, 76).

SCI patients use different patterns during walking with orthosis, which include (91, 92):

a)   Four- points gait pattern
b)   Swing through gait pattern
c)   Swing to gait pattern
d)   Drag –to pattern
e)   Reciprocal gait pattern

However, the two most common used methods are swing through and reciprocal gait patterns.

5.2   Swing through gait

This method of transportation is selected by the patients who have lesion level at T_9 or lower. This is the quickest form of locomotion, which can be selected by those patients. The arms and crutches move forward and then the body swing forward. For those SCI individuals who have spasticity of abdominals muscles, this style is not useful. The strength of elbow extensors is important to lift the body weight during swing phase. Figure 5.1 shows this style of walking (92, 93).

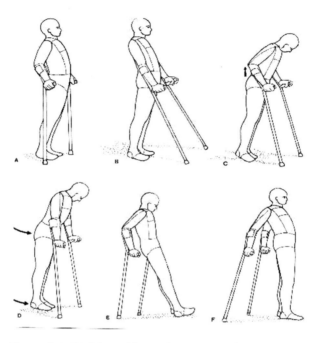

Figure 5.1: Walking with a swing throgh gait pattern (93)

5.3 Reciprocal Gait Pattern

Reciprocal gait is defined as a pattern in which the legs move separately and alternatively. In this gait pattern the subject places one foot in front of the other foot in the manner that one leg is always bearing weight (55, 60). This form of walking requires three actions, which include:

 a) Removing the swing leg from the ground

b) Moving the swing leg hip joint from extension to flexion

c) Moving the trunk forwards over the stance leg

The paraplegic subjects walk with reciprocal gait pattern with new HKAFO orthoses such as with the HGO, LSU RGO and ARGO orthoses. During normal walking, extension of the hip joint is achieved by muscular force however, during paraplegic walking this force must be injected into the system through the arms and crutches. The role of lattismusDorsi muscle is more important and noticeable than that of other muscles to transmit the force of the crutch and the upper limb to the pelvis. Other muscles such as pectoralis major, deltoid and trapeziuses are active to stabilize the shoulder joint and to help the lattismusDorsi to transmit the force to the pelvis. As soon as the swing leg clears the ground, it starts to swing forward to the midline by the effect of gravity. Then the swing leg moves beyond the midline by inertial effect (76). The gait of the SCI individuals with reciprocal gait pattern with the HGO orthosis is divided into different stages as follows:

Stage 1:

This stage is the same as heel contact during normal walking. The crutch of the stance leg (Right) is positioned forward and the left crutch is behind. This stage is the beginning stage of walking (figure 5.2).

Stage 2:

In this stage the majority of the body weight is applied on the right foot and the left foot is ready to start swing phase. The right crutch is in the front of the right foot and the left crutch is positioned slightly ahead of the left foot. It should be mentioned that the force applied on the left crutch is more than that applied on the right crutch. The extensors of the elbow and shoulder joints on the left side stabilize the joints and help the subjects to lift the body weight from the left side and to transmit it to the contra lateral side. The amount of flexion of the right hip joint decreases and it starts to move through the uphill phase by the help of the backward directed left crutch force. The function of some muscles such as left and right shoulder joint stabilizers, left latismusDorsi, triceps and pectoralis major is significant in this stage of walking with the HGO orthosis (61, 76). Figure 5.2 shows some events that are taking place in this stage during walking with HGO orthosis.

Stage 3:

This stage is the same as foot flat in the gait of the normal subjects. The vertical force applied on the left crutch is significantly more than that of the right crutch. The left crutch is completely fixed on the ground and the force of latismusDorsi and other shoulder extensors are transmitted to the right side as the main force for pelvic forward motion. As in the previous stage the role of shoulder joint extensors in the left side is very important. The event which is taking place in this stage is shown in figure 5.2.

Stage 4:

The crutch on the left side is removed from the ground and the force applied on it decreases to zero. In contrast the force applied on the right crutch increases. The right side of the pelvis starts to move to the downhill phase and the right hip joint starts to extend. In this stage the left leg is in the swing phase. The activity of some muscles such as, triceps and shoulder girdle muscle is more significant in the right side than in the left side. The structural rigidity of the HGO resists the adduction moments applied on the right leg. This stage is shown in figure 5.2.

Stage 5:

This stage is the same as toe off in the gait of a normal subject. The weight of the body will be transmitted to the left foot at the end of this stage. The forward motion of the right hip joint is significant, due to forward moment gained from the downhill phase. Some muscles such as triceps and shoulder depressors start to contract in order to control the force applied on the right crutch (61, 76). This stage is shown in figure 5.2.

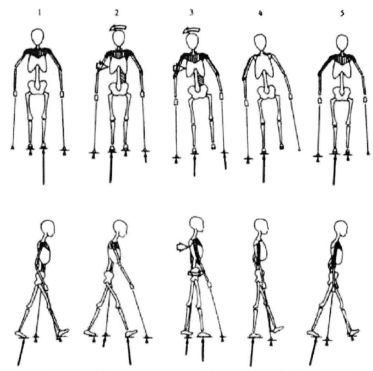

Figure 5.2: The different stages of walking with HGO orthosis(55)

5.4   Temporal gait parameters

The temporal gait parameters of SCI individuals during walking with an orthosis depends on the pattern of the gait, selected by those patients and also on the type of orthosis used. In the research by Melis et al (1999), the temporal gait parameters of 10 incomplete SCI patients, with lesion levels between C_5 and T_{12}, were collected during

87

walking with different assistive devices, without orthosis. The mean walking speed for the walker users varied from 0.05 to 0.29 m/s however, for the crutch users it was between 0.3 and 0.8 m/s. The walker which was used by the participants was a common one with four rubber tips. Table 5.1 shows the mean values of the temporal gait parameters according to the research done by Melis et al (1999).

Parameters	Walking (speed m/s)	Cadence (Steps/min)	Step length (m)	Stance/swing ratio	Max. Crutch force % of BW
Walker users	0.17 ±0.04	30 ±13	0.3 ±0.11	From 73/27 to 95/5	74% ±395
Crutch users	From 0.3 to 0.8	From 42 to 89.3	From 0.43 to 0.67	From 69/31 to 74/26	From 15% to 50%

Table 5.1: Some parameters in walking with swing through gait pattern with crutch and walker (94)

The biomechanical parameters of the normal subjects, who wore a pair of KAFOs, and the paraplegic subjects, who used the same orthosis differ from each other's during walking with swing to gait and swing through gait patterns. In research done by Noreau et al (1995) the temporal gait parameters of the normal subjects walked with a pair of KAFOs and the paraplegic subjects used the same orthosis were measured. The paraplegic subjects walked faster than normal subjects who walked with orthoses however, their walking performances reduced significantly during walking with swing to gait pattern in contrast to swing through gait pattern (95). Table 5.2 shows some results of this research.

Parameters	Normal subjects*		Paraplegic subjects Swing through gait		Paraplegic subjects Swing to gait
	Slow	Fast	Slow	Fast	Combined
Velocity (m/s)	40.4 ±5.7	57.5 ±13.2	41.7 ±5.2	59.9 ±9.8	23.4 ±6.6
Cadence (steps/min)	59 ±6	70 ±10	67 ±7	79 ±7	88 ±3.2
Stride length (m)	1.34 ±0.15	1.6 ± 0.15	1.23 ±0.11	1.5 ±0.17	0.53 ±0.18
Stance phase percentage	78.8 ±4.5	74 ±4.2	70.7 ±5	64.6 ± 5.9	83.9 ±6.4

Table 5.2: Some results of the research done by Noreau(95)

The normal subjects walked with a pair of KAFOs

The cadence, walking speed, stride length and stance phase duration differs during walking with reciprocal gait and swing through gait pattern. Slavens et al (2007) examined the temporal distance parameters of SCI patients which walked with reciprocal gait and swing through gait patterns. The subject population included three girls and two boys with the age between 8 and 12 years and with a myelodysplasia with a level of lesion at L_3 and L_4. They found that swing through gait produced a high walking speed and cadence. Table 5.3 shows the results of the research done by Slavens et al.

The gait parameters during walking with reciprocal gait pattern also depend on the orthosis. Walking speed during walking with the RGO and the HGO orthoses is nearly 0.3 (8, 96). Table 5.4 shows some gait parameters during walking with the RGO, HGO and A RGO orthoses.

Temporal Parameters	Walking speed (m/s)	Cadence (Steps/min)	Step length (m)	Stance duration (Sec)
Reciprocal gait	0.39	67.12	0.66	0.66
Swing through gait	0.59	75.43	0.86	0.63

Table 5.3: The result of the research done by Slavens(97)

Parameters	RGO	A RGO	HGO
Cadence	35	37	37
Stride length	1.02	0.99	0.98
Velocity (m/sec)	0.3	0.31	0.3
Stance phase %	67	67	67

Table 5.4: Gait parameters of a paraplegic subject during walking with three different orthoses (8)

5.5 Kinematic parameters during paraplegic walking

A paraplegic individual walking with a swing through gait, with KAFO orthosis has almost the same hip joint flexion as that in normal subject (35 degrees). The excursion of the shoulder joint in the sagittal plane, which is approximately 40 degrees does not vary significantly between normal subjects and paraplegic subjects during walking with a swing through gait pattern. Since the stance phase of the crutch is longer in paraplegic subjects in contrast to that in normal subject so flexion of the shoulder occurs with a little delay in those patients (95). In their research 8 paraplegic subjects with 9 normal subjects were selected and were trained to walk with a pair of KAFOs.

Parameters	RGO	Steeper RGO	HGO
Hip joint flexion	15	12	16
Hip joint extension	33	35	21
Hip joint abduction	3	0	9
Hip joint adduction	8	10	7

Table 5.5: Hip joint range of motion during walking with different orthoses (8)

Parameters	RGO	Steeper RGO	HGO
Motion in sagittal plane	16	17	11
Motion in coronal plane	16	17	12
Motion in transverse plane	23	26	33

Table 5.6: Pelvic motions in the different planes during walking with different orthoses (8)

SCI individuals who walked with a walker have a forward flexion in trunk during entire the gait cycle. According to the results of the research done by Melis et al (1999), trunk flexion varied between 10 and 40 degrees during walking with crutch (94). In this research, which 10 subjects with incomplete SCI participated, the mean value of hip joint flexion extension excursion during walking with a walker was a little more than that during walking with a crutch. In contrast those walked with a crutch had more extension in the trunk and were able to extend their hip joint during stance phase (94).

During walking with a HGO orthosis, a paraplegic's hip joint flexes more than that during walking with the RGO and ARGO orthoses. In contrast, the hip joint extends less in an HGO orthosis compared with the other two orthoses. The motion of the pelvis with HGO differs from that in the other two orthoses, it has less motion in coronal and

91

sagittal planes in contrast to other orthoses (8). Tables 5.5 and 5.6 show the hip and pelvic angles for a paraplegic individual walking with HGO, RGO and ARGO orthoses.

5.6 Force applied on the crutch and foot during walking with orthoses with various walking styles

The magnitude of the forces applied on the crutch and foot during walking of paraplegic subjects depends not only on the pattern of walking, but also on the orthosis used. The magnitude of the anteroposterior shear and the vertical forces applied on the crutch during walking with swing through gait is slightly greater than that in walking with swing to gait. However, there is no difference between the mediolateral force applied on the crutch in walking with the two styles (98).

In the research conducted by Slavens et al, the force applied on the crutch was between 44.7 and 45.1 % of BW with a reciprocal gait pattern and between 55.62 and 57.2 % of BW during walking with a swing through gait pattern (97).

Major et al (1981) carried out a research to show the magnitude of the forces applied on the foot and crutch in walking of a paraplegic subject with the HGO orthosis. According to the results of this study, the magnitude of the vertical ground reaction force applied on the right foot and left crutch were 90% and 22% of BW, respectively at initial contact. At foot flat 65% of the BW was applied on the right leg, compared to 35% of the left crutch. The maximum magnitude of the vertical force was applied on the foot just prior to toe off (110% of BW). The peak of the mediolateral force applied on the crutches during walking with the HGO was 5 % of BW.

While, in the research done by Nene and Major (1987) with nine paraplegic subjects with lesion between levels T_4 and T_9 the maximum values of the vertical force applied on the foot varied between 29% and 98% of BW, compared to 40% of BW applied on the crutch. In further research done in Milan University by Ferrarin and his co-workers (99) the biomechanical parameters of five HGO users with lesion levels between T_1 and T_{10} and also a matched control group were assessed during walking. The results of this research showed that there was a significant difference between the duration of stance and swing phases between normal subjects and paraplegics and also between skilled and unskilled Parawalker users. The results of this research are shown in table 5.7.

Patients	Maximum vertical force applied on the foot (% of BW)	Maximum vertical force applied on the crutch (% of BW)	Foot vertical force impulse (% of total) (Ns)	Crutch vertical force impulse (% of total) (Ns)
Skilled	78.4%	29.6%	71.2%	28.8%
Unskilled	104.2%	28.85	79.4%	20.6%

Table 5.7:The kinetic parameters of the walking with the HGO (99)

According to the research by Tashman et al (1995), the maximum values of the ground reaction force applied on the limb and crutch was 83% and 33% of BW during walking with the RGO orthosis. The hip joint range of motion (flexion extension) in this research was nearly 25 degrees. The magnitude of the mediolateral shear forces applied on the foot was minimal. In another research project carried out by Ijzerman et al (1997) the peak of the crutch force of five paraplegic subjects (with lesion between levels T_4 and T_{12}) during walking with the ARGO orthosis with various degrees of abduction was

93

measured. According to the results of this research the maximum values of the crutch force varied between 0.33 to 0.49% of BW.

It can be concluded from the above mentioned research that the force applied on the crutch during walking with a reciprocal gait pattern is significantly less than that with swing through gait and swing to gait patterns. Moreover, the amount of the force differed between skilled and unskilled subjects.

CHAPTER 6: ASSESSMENT OF THE AVAILABLE ORTHOSES USED FOR STANDING AND WALKING OF PARAPLEGIC SUBJECTS

6.1 Introduction

A variety of orthoses have been designed to enable SCI to stand and walk again however, none of them are without any problems. The important point is that the appropriate orthosis must be selected according to the level of lesion and also of the ability of the subjects to walk. There are some methods used to assess the performance of SCI individuals during standing and walking with different orthoses. According to Stallard and Major (1998) the main factors for assessment of the orthosis include:

a) Independency of patients in using the orthosis

b) Energy cost of walking with the orthosis

c) Cosmesis

d) Mechanical reliability

e) System cost

For the cosmesis, other parameters such as the style of walking and degree to which the orthosis can be seen under the clothing were considered. The other parameters that can be used for evaluation of the orthosis are as follow (100):

a) Efficiency of the orthosis during walking

b) Ease of application

c) Assistive devices required for walking

d) Cosmesis of walking and of the orthosis

The efficiency of orthosis was defined as the amount of energy consumption during walking with the orthosis. However, Whittle et al (1991) also selected other parameters to compare the performance of 22 paraplegic subjects who walked with the HGO and RGO orthoses. They considered some factors such as the facilities and time required to fabricate the orthosis, the time required to train the subject, gait parameters, the cosmesis of the orthosis itself and the cost of the final orthosis and training cost. The gait parameters which were selected by different investigators to compare the performance of the orthoses include (7, 8):

a) Cadence, stride length, walking velocity, percentage of the stance phase in contrast to the total gait time
b) Pattern of movement
c) Hip joint range of motion in the sagittal and coronal planes
d) Pelvic angular motion and translations

The stability of the subject during quiet standing and doing hand tasks was another parameter which was selected by different investigators (101-103). Other parameters such as the weight of the orthosis are not important factors for ambulation of the patients with orthosis because it is not required to lift the orthosis completely from the ground by patients during reciprocal walking (9). Further research to support the concept that the weight of orthosis does not affect the performance of the subject during walking was published by Corcoran et al (1970).

Therefore in order to evaluate a new designed orthosis, parameters such as standing stability during quiet standing and while undertaking different hand functions, energy consumption during walking and gait parameters should be measured. Other parameters such as the cosmesis of the orthosis and the style of walking, and mechanical reliability of the orthosis also influence the interest of the subjects to use an orthosis.

96

6.2 Standing stability

Stability during standing is achieved by a complex process which involves the coordination activities of multiple sensory, motor and biomechanical components. In normal subjects stability is maintained by coordinated motions which occurred at the knee, hip and ankle joints. The role of the muscles which surround these joints is very important and effective to maintain the stability during standing. In order to have good balance the COG of body must be within the base of support. During normal standing, some strategies such as head movement strategies, trunk strategies, hip and ankle strategies can be used in order to maintain stability (104). However, in SCI individuals these strategies cannot be used and the amount of stability depends on the external support, which is achieved by using the orthosis. The structural stiffness of the orthosis is an important factor which increases the amount of stability during paraplegic standing (61).

There are two different assessment methods which are used to check the amount of standing stability. The first method which was developed by Romberg at the beginning of nineteen century was based on the amount of body sway under opened and closed eyes conditions. The difference between body sway during standing with eyes open and closed represents the functional performance of the somatosensory system which controls the stability. By using force platform technology the researchers are more able to measure the postural sway to analyse the stability in different positions. The second approach was to check the stability when an unexpected force was applied on the body.

6.2.1 Assessment methods to evaluate the standing stability during quiet standing based on the force plate data

To assess the amount of stability the location of the Centre of Pressure (COP) is measured during a period of time. Many of the parameters mentioned in the literature for stability analysis are based on COP location change with respect to time. The following parameters used by different investigators to measure the standing stability.

a)   The COP path length (102)

b)   The COP sway excursion in the mediolateral and anteroposterior directions (101, 105)

c)   The average speed of the COP change (106)

d)   The location of the COP in contrast to the base of support (101)

e)   Mean amplitude of the COP sway in mediolateral and anteroposterior planes (107)

f)   Measuring the force applied on the force plate (108)

g)   Hip joint motion in the standing position (109)

h)   The amount of the force applied on the crutch during walking (101)

Amongst different parameters which can be used for measuring the stability during quiet standing, using the excursions of the COP in the mediolateral and anteroposterior planes has been used by many researchers. These excursions are easy to use and have good validity and repeatability in showing the standing stability (105, 106). Moreover, the use of the force applied on the crutch in order to analyse the standing stability of the paraplegic subjects, has been recommended (101).

6.2.2 Standing stability during hand function

The stability test of paraplegics and normal subjects during standing with an orthosis was carried out during quiet standing in many research projects. However, the functional stability test is another important factor which was considered only in a few studies. The Jebson test of the hand function is one of the standard tests used for analysis of the stability during hand function. This test was extended to include tasks which required vertical reaching and crossing the midline while standing and represents both fine and gross motor skills. Triolo et al (1993) evaluated the functional stability of 69 able bodies and 2 paraplegic subjects. Subjects undertook the following tasks during standing:

a)   Move small objects on countertop
b)   Lift objects to low shelf
c)   Lift objects from low shelf
d)   Push objects from dominate side

The time required to do these tasks was the main factor selected for final analysis. The results of the SCI patients showed that this test is very patient dependant, because one of the participants did the test in the normal limit but, the second performed poorly. The results of this research showed that more work must be done to check reliability and repeatability for both normal and paraplegic subjects.

The functional stability of paraplegic subjects while undertaking different hand tasks was measured by other investigators. They measured some parameters such as, the excursions of the COP in the mediolateral and anteroposterior planes, the time required to undertake various hand tasks and the force applied on the crutch (101, 102).

6.3 Evaluation of the walking performances by measuring the amount of energy consumption during ambulation

The amount of consumed energy during walking is one of the important parameters which are selected routinely for evaluation of the performance of different assistive devices. Measuring the energy consumption during various activities based on indirect calorimetry, which is based on the assumption that all energy releasing reactions in human body ultimately depends on the utilization of the oxygen. For measuring the amount of oxygen during walking the following methods were used by various investigators, which include:

a) Douglas bag (110)

b) Mobile Automatic Metabolic Analyser (MAMA) (111)

c) Cosmed K2 b2 gas analyser (112)

d) Cosmed K4 b2 gas analyser (113, 114)

From the above procedures, the use of Cosmed K4 gas analyser is more reliable and easier to use than others. Measuring the rate of oxygen consumption is a good way to assess the energy used during walking, however the instruments are cumbersome to wear and also may not be available in all clinics. Using these systems also restricts the abilities of the participants and indirectly influences their performances. This involves using a nose clip by subjects and breathing through a snugly fixed mask. However, in clinical situations involving different persons with physical handicap, using these methods is not very practical and it is better that other methods used instead (84, 86).

Heart rate is an accurate estimation of the oxygen consumption and is a simple and easy to use parameter in any conditions (86). It has been stated by several authors that apparently there does not seem to be a close relationship between energy expenditure and heart rate. But it is clear that the main part of the energy in our body is supplied by aerobic oxidate reaction, in which oxygen is the main part of the process. The oxygen is carried by the blood and the blood is pumped into muscles by the heart. The harder our muscles work the more oxygen is used and more blood is required, so the heart must work harder and the rate of breathing would be increased. Therefore, it is clear that there is a noticeable relationship between heart rate and energy and oxygen consumption (115).

The relationship between heart rate and oxygen consumption was evaluated in the different research studies. In research carried out by Rose et al (1989), the mean value of the correlation coefficient was 0.98±0.2 and 0.99±0.1 for normal and CP participants (18 normal and 13 CP patients), respectively. Moreover, in research done by Goosery and Tolfrey (2004), which was done on trained female wheelchair athletes, the correlation coefficient between heart rate and oxygen consumption was 0.973. Bar-On and Nene (1990) were other investigators that measured the correlation between the heart rate and oxygen consumption in paraplegic subjects with various lesions between levels T_3 and T_{10}. Their heart rate and their oxygen consumption were monitored during various activities. The results of this study showed a high correlation coefficient between heart rate and oxygen consumption during activities. For patients with lesion level between T_3 and T_6 the co-efficient of correlation was 0.7824 and for those with lesion level from T_7 to T_{10} it was 0.8592. The patients with high spinal cord injury level miss the control of para-sympatic centre which is supposed to be around T_4 (116).

6.3.1 Heart Rate per Distance Walked

Heart rate expressed per distance walked indicates the energy economy (84). The following equation was used to check the Energy Expenditure Index (EEI, beats per meter) (117):

$$EEI \ (beats/metre) = \frac{heart \ rate \ during \ exercise - heart \ rate \ during \ resting \ (beats/min)}{Walking \ speed \ (metre/min)}$$

Eq. 2.4

This equation has been used mostly in various research projects to evaluate the efficiency of different orthoses, which is also named as Physiological Cost Index (PCI). In the research carried out by Rose et al (1990) the amount of oxygen consumed during walking and heart rate per meter were compared in 12 children with cerebral palsy and 18 normal subjects. They found that the curve of the heart rate per metre and oxygen consumed per metre was similar for both groups. It was also shown that the mean value of EEI in disabled group was significantly more than that in the normal group.

The results of the different researches carried out on normal and paraplegic subjects showed that the PCI has high test retest reliability (0.843-0.944). Moreover, it was shown that PCI is an easy to use, valid and reliable measure of energy expenditure and it is a good factor to check the efficiency of any orthoses and to evaluate any locomotion disabilities. However, some researchers such as Ijzerman et al (1999) recommended that since the number of patients participated in the research related to SCI subjects is limited, it is recommended to use other variable to have strong statistical results.

6.4 Assessment the level of independency in using an orthosis by SCI subject

The level of independency in using of any orthoses is scored according to a five points scale modified from functional independence major. Those points include (118):

a)   Independent (no help or assistance)

b)   Stand by assistance (no physical assistance from helper but only verbal prompting)

c)   Minimal assistance (patients do 75% of the task themselves)

d)   Moderate assistance (patients do a task themselves between 25 % to 75%)

e)   Maximal assistance

The other important factor to check the comfort of the patients in using an orthosis is the time required for donning and doffing the orthosis.

CHAPTER 7: EVALUATION OF THE AVAILABLE ORTHOSES WHICH ARE USED FOR SCI'S WALKING AND STANDING

7.1 Introduction

Different types of orthoses, mechanical, hybrid and externally powered have been designed for paraplegic subjects however, many of them have not been produced commercially. The performance of the well-known orthoses is mentioned in the following section.

7.2 Evaluation of the performance of paraplegics during walking with AFO and KAFO orthoses

There is no doubt that many paraplegic subjects cannot use AFO orthoses, since many of them have knee extensor paralysis and the AFO cannot provide enough support for this joint. The Vannini_Rizzolo stabilizing orthosis is one of the specifically designed AFO orthoses for paraplegic subjects. However, a number of contraindications were considered in selecting the patients to use this orthosis. The contraindication parameters which were considered in that research were: contractions of the lower limbs joints, instability of the knee joint due to laxity of the ligaments, overweight by more than 20% of ideal weight, instability of the spinal column and any problems in the cardiovascular system (50).

From the 58 patients with lesion levels between T_2 and L_5 who participated in this study, 29 patients were selected for final analysis according to those above contraindication factors. They were asked to walk with a comfortable speed. The distance ambulated with the boot differed from 1.524 to 152.4 meter, and averaged 26.03 meter.

The energy consumption of a group of paraplegic subjects (22 patients) was measured by Waters and Lunsford (1985). The results of this research showed that the mean values of walking speed and heart rate during ambulation with orthosis were 26±16 m/min, 131±24 beats/min, respectively. Some results of this research are shown in table 7.1.

Parameters	Heart rate (beats/min)	Speed (m/min)	Oxygen rate (ml/kg/min)	Oxygen cost (ml/kg/m)
Mean value	131± 24	26± 16	13.8 ±4.8	0.73 ±0.49

Table 7.1:Some results based on the research carried out by Waters and Lunsford (1985)

The performance of paraplegic subjects during walking with KAFO orthoses was evaluated by many investigators. In the research carried out by Huang et al (1979), the amount of energy consumption during walking with a Craig-Scott orthosis was measured on 8 paraplegic subjects with lesion level between T_4 and T_{12}. In the resting state, the average O_2 consumption was 0.061 ml/sec/kg and the mean energy cost was 17.12 cal/min/kg however, they were 0.1867 ml/s/kg and 52.96 cal/min/kg, respectively during ambulation. The results of this research showed that the oxygen consumption during walking with this orthosis was three times more than that during resting position (111).

Other research work was carried out by Merkel et al (1984) to evaluate the efficiency of two KAFO orthoses in standing and walking of paraplegic patients. Eight paraplegics with lesion levels between C_7 and T_{12} participated in this study. They walked with a Scott-Craig KAFO and single-stopped long-leg KAFO with walker and crutches. The speed of walking with the Scott- Craig and walker was 8.8±5.8 m/min in contrast to 6.3± 2.45 m/min for single-stopped KAFO orthosis (plantar flexion fixed). However, it didn't differ when the subjects used crutches as their assistive device. The results of this study showed that the Scott-Craig was a more energy efficient orthosis than the single-stopped long-leg KAFO in walking, by 25% to 34% depending on the type of the selected assistive device (119). The results of another research done by Lehman et al (1969) showed that the performance of subjects using KAFO orthoses with anterior and posterior ankle stops was significantly better than those who walked with KAFO orthoses with free dorsiflexion motion.

In conclusion, many paraplegic subjects cannot use AFO orthosis for walking. This orthosis is suitable for SCI subjects with a lower lesion of the spinal cord and those who have some knee extensor power. However, many paraplegic subjects can use KAFO orthoses for standing and walking. The performance of SCI subjects with Scott-Craig KAFOs with fixed ankle joints is better than other available KAFO orthoses.

7.3 Evaluation of the performance of paraplegics walking with HKAFO orthoses

Amongst various HKAFO orthoses designed for paraplegic subjects, the HGO, RGO and ARGO orthoses are the orthoses which have been produced commercially and used by the patients. The results of the research to evaluate the performance of the SCI individuals in using the HKAFO orthoses are as follows.

7.3.1 Evaluation of the functional performance of SCI individuals walking with HGO orthosis

106

The energy cost of ten paraplegic subjects, with complete spinal cord lesion between T_4 and T_9, in walking with the HGO orthosis was measured by Nene and Patrick (1989). They walked with crutch and with a self-selected comfortable speed. The average walking speed varied from 0.133 to 0.349 m/s, the mean value was 0.214 m/s. The mean values of energy cost and energy consumption in walking with the HGO were 16 J/kg/m and 3.1 J/kg/s, respectively.

In other research work carried out by Moore and Stallard (1991), the performance of the HGO orthosis was evaluated on 50 paraplegic subjects with a lesion ranging from level L_1 to T_3 by using direct interview. The main criterion in selecting the patients was using the orthosis for at least 6 months. The results of this study showed that 64% of the HGO users were still using their devices. It should be mentioned that the mean time of review follow up after orthosis supply was 34.4 months. Nearly 78% of them used their orthoses, independently. Approximately 20% of users reported that their orthosis had some functional use for them. According to the results of this research, using the orthosis in driving or using public transportation systems were the main problems associated with the users.

In another research carried out by Stallard and Major (1995) the effect of increasing the lateral stiffness of the HGO orthosis on the gait performance of SCI individuals was evaluated by the introduction of the Parawalker 89. The amount of energy consumption of three participants with lesion levels between T_8 and L_1 was analyzed by using PCI. The results of this study showed that PCI was reduced when subjects walking with Parawalker 89 from 1.4 to 0.98 (30% reduction). Moreover, in other research work, they showed that increasing the lateral stiffness of the orthosis increased the walking speed between 13 and 83% and decreased energy cost between 12 and 42% (61).

107

The performance of the paraplegic subjects in walking with the Parawaker 89 is significantly better than older versions of this orthosis, because its lateral stiffness is more than the previous orthoses. Nearly two third of paraplegic subjects used this orthosis only inside home and for therapeutic purposes. They had some problems when they used their orthosis in the community. The problems with driving and using public transportation systems were the two most common issues mentioned by the users.

7.3.2 Evaluation the functional performance of SCI individuals walking with the RGO orthosis

The first research on the performance of the SCI subjects while walking with the RGO was done by Douglas et al (1983). They mentioned in this research that the brace was successfully fitted on 138 patients having some disorders such as spina bifida, paraplegia, cerebral palsy, multiple sclerosis, muscular dystrophy, and sacral agenesis. It was found that adults, paralyzed from spinal cord injury accepted this orthosis because it was more energy efficient than the conventional orthoses. They were able to walk 304.8 meter with no more than two 30 seconds rest periods.

Energy consumption in children with myelomeningoclyle during walking with the traditional HKAFO and the RGO was evaluated by Cuddeford et al (1997). This research was done on 26 children with myelomeningoclyle, which 15 of them selected RGO and 11 of them used the HKAFO orthosis. The average velocity of the RGO users was 0.27 m/s compared to 0.68 m/s for those who used the HKAFO orthosis. There was a significant difference between the energy costs during walking with two orthoses. Some results of this research are shown in table 7.2. There was no information regarding the gait parameters in this research however, since the subjects walked with swing through gait pattern with the HKAFO orthosis, more force applied on their upper limb in contrast to that in walking with the RGO orthosis.

108

Orthosis	Energy consumption (VO$_2$/kg/min)	Energy cost (VO$_2$/kg/meter)	Walking velocity (m/s)
RGO	11.44 (±1.85)	0.81 (±0.34)	0.27 (±0.11)
Traditional HKAFO	21.1 (±3.08)	0.54 (±0.12)	0.68 (±0.20)

Table 7.2:The results of the research done by Cudderford et al (1997)

Dall (2004) carried out research to check the magnitude of the forces and then calculated the moments of the hip joint applied on the front and back cables of the LSU RGO orthosis during paraplegic walking. To measure the cable tension, special transducers were embedded between the cables and the hip joint attachments, figure 7.1. Six paraplegic subjects with lesion levels between C_5/C_6 and T_{11}/T_{12} participated in this study. The magnitude of the forces and moments of both cables was evaluated during swing and stance phases.

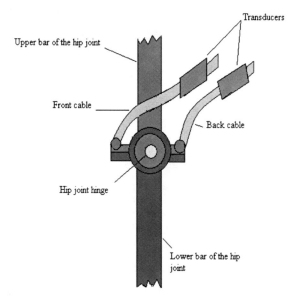

Figure 7.1: The sketch of the hip joint of the RGO orthosis with transducers used in the research carried out by Dall et al.

The result of this study showed that the role of the back cable is more important than that of the front cable during walking especially during double limb support period. In four of six subjects the <u>front</u> cable was not used (the force recorded was zero). In the other two subjects the moments produced by this cable varied between 0 and 5 Nm.

In double limb support phase, the <u>back</u> cable was in tension between 97% and 100% of the stance phase; but it was in tension from 40% to 90% of the swing phase for all subjects. The maximum moment generated by this cable, according to the result of this research was in the double limb support and it varied from 12 to 35 Nm. In contrast it was between 8 and 14 Nm in the swing phase of gait. The flexor moment around the hip joint in the normal subjects as cited by Dall from Winter (1991) is around 40 Nm, so the moment applied on the front cable in swing phase is very low to produce any motion during swing phase (83, 120).

It was expected that the reciprocal cables in the RGO orthosis transmit the motion from one side to other side. This means that the extension of one side produces flexion in the contralateral side (48, 65). However, the results of the research done by Dall et al (1999) showed that the tension developed in the front cable is significantly small. However, the back cable is in the tension for the most parts of the stance and swing phases. Moreover, the tension developed in the back cable is not sufficiently high to force the legs to move.

7.3.3 Evaluation of the functional performance of SCI individuals walking with the ARGO orthosis

The first research which focused on the performance of a paraplegic subject during walking with the ARGO orthosis was carried out by Jefferson and Whittle (1990). The results of this research showed that the performance of the ARGO wasn't as good as the HGO orthosis. The results of this study have already bean shown in tables 5.5 and 5.6 and discussed.

In other research carried out by Ijzerman et al (1997b) the effects of frontal alignment in the ARGO was evaluated on the gait performance of paraplegic subjects. Five paraplegic subjects with lesion from levels T_4 to T_{12} were selected for this study. The results of this study showed that incorporating an abduction angle in the alignment of the ARGO increases the functional performance of the orthosis. Table 7.3 shows some results which were collected from this study.

111

Orthosis	CTFI (N.s)	CPF (N/BW) in stance phase	CPF (N/BW) in swing phase	Walking speed (m/s)
ARGO (6 degrees adduction)	0.59± 0.12	0.39 ±0.05	0.43± 0.02	0.29± 0.09
ARGO with 0 degrees abduction	0.57± 0.12	0.36± 0.04	0.4 ±0.02	0.28± 0.09
ARGO with 3 degrees abduction	0.56± 0.13	0.36± 0.04	0.41 ±0.03	0.28± 0.11
ARGO with 6 degrees abduction	0.59± 0.21	0.33± 0.07	0.49± 0.07	0.26± 0.11

Table 7.3:The results of the research done by Ijzerman et al (1997b)

CTFI = Crutch Time Force Integral, CPF= Crutch Peak Force

The effect of the Bowden cable of the ARGO on the walking performances of paraplegic subjects was analyzedby Ijzerman et al (1997a). Six paraplegic subjects were selected for this study with lesion levels between T_4 and T_{12}. The average walking speed with the ARGO and NRGO were 0.24 and 0.23 m/s, respectively. The mean value of the oxygen cost in walking with the ARGO was 1.55 ml/m/kg compared with 1.63 ml/m/kg during walking with the NRGO orthosis. The mean difference in oxygen cost in walking with the NRGO varied from 25% higher to 17% lower than that of the ARGO. There was no significant difference between the performances of the two orthoses during walking of the participants. For participants with higher lesion level, the oxygen consumption in the NRGO was nearly 40% higher than the ARGO. The walking speed of the participants with the NRGO was slower than that of the ARGO.

However, for those with lower lesion level, their performance was better during walking with the NRGO orthosis. According to the results of this research, paraplegics with higher lesion levels could benefits less from the NRGO orthosis than those with lower lesion level. For higher lesion levels the motion of the hip joint must be more limited in order to increase the stability of the participants during walking. The results of this research showed that the effect of using reciprocal cables in theARGO orthosison the walking performance is not as important as expected.

In other research carried out by Baardman et al (1997) the influence of using Bowden cable in the ARGO on standing of paraplegic subjects was evaluated. Six paraplegic subjects participated in this study. The standing performances of the participants with two types of the ARGO, with removed Bowden cable (A_GO) and the ARGO, was analyzed after 4 weeks training programme. There was no difference between the functional performances of the two orthoses in standing of the subjects. The mean COP anteroposterior ranges were 37.94 and 35.22 millimetres for the A_GO and the ARGO orthoses, respectively. In the mediolateral direction the ranges were 34.53 mm for the A_GO and 41.72 mm for the ARGO orthosis. According to the results of this research, using the back cable in the ARGO doesn't have a significant influence on the standing stability (101).

The effect of lesion level on the gait performance of the SCI subjects was examined by Kawashima et al (2003). Ten paraplegic subjects with a complete injury at thoracic levels (T_5 toT_{12}) were selected for this study. All participants underwent 10 weeks of training using the ARGO. The mean walking speed of the participants during walking with the ARGO, according to the results of this research was 19.88 m/min. The results of this research showed that the slower gait speed and higher energy cost of the patients with a high lesion level can be attributed to the limited range of motion of the hip joint. The mean values of the hip joint range of motion was 45 degrees (121).

In summary, the review of the above three papers indicated that the performance of paraplegic subjects in walking with the ARGO orthosis, aligned in a slight abduction, was significantly better than that with the orthosis without abduction. The effect of the reciprocal cable on the standing stability and gait performance is not as supposed to be. There was no difference between the energy consumption of the subjects in walking with the ARGO orthosis with and without cable. However, it can be concluded that SCI subjects with a higher level of lesion should use the orthosis with the cable.

7.4   Evaluation the functional performance of the SCI individuals during walking with the other types of orthoses

The HGO, RGO, and ARGO orthoses are three commonly used orthoses for paraplegic subjects. Some researchers have tried to design some orthoses to improve the function however, the final results was not successful. The design of some mechanical orthosis such as the WO and MLO orthoses improved the donning and doffing of the orthoses by the subjects however, it decreased the function of the subjects during walking (118). Using some mechanisms, such as the sliding mechanism to decrease the height discrepancy between the hip joints (mechanical and anatomical ones) may improve the performance of the subjects during walking on the level surface however, it decreases the performance of the paraplegics in walking on uneven surface (70). Moreover, it decreased the cosmesis of the orthosis and the willingness of the subjects to use the orthosis. Using other types of mechanisms such as, attaching the hip and ankle joints to each other, had no effects on improving the function of the orthosis however, it obviously decreased the cosmesis of the orthosis (72).

The performance of the externally powered orthoses is not as good as the commonly used mechanical orthoses. Moreover, the patients have to use the orthosis which is heavy and more difficult to donn and doff independently (64, 113, 121). Sometimes they have to charge the batteries regularly which take a lot of time and need special facilities (122).

In the hybrid orthosis (combination of the mechanical orthosis with functional electrical stimulation as discussed before) the main emphasis of the designers were to improve the function of the orthosis by using knee flexion, ankle and knee motions and by increasing the stiffness of the orthosis. The results of different research showed that in some of them the performance of the subjects did not improve significantly, however the style of walking improved as the patients had knee flexion during swing phase (82, 123, 124). Although using FES with the HGO orthosis improved the performance of the subjects in using the orthosis however, they have some problems which include (61):

a)   They had problems with using the electrodes in suitable locations
b)   They achieved inconsistent stimulation
c)   Donning and doffing the orthosis with stimulation electrodes was very time consuming
d)   Cross stimulation of abdominal muscles occurred

In conclusion, the performance of paraplegic subjects in using commonly used orthoses such as the HGO, RGO and ARGO orthoses is better than the hybrid and externally powered orthoses.

7.5 Comparison between the different transportation mechanisms selected by the SCI individuals

The main transportation methods which are selected by SCI individuals are using orthosis and wheelchairs. Both of them have some advantages and disadvantages. Although these subjects have to use orthoses in order to maintain their health and to improve the functions of various organs, they may prefer to use wheelchairs as a main mode of the locomotion.

7.5.1 Comparison between the various orthoses used by the SCI individuals

As was mentioned in the previous part of this thesis, a variety of orthoses have been designed for SCI subjects in order to stand and walk. However, their walking performance significantly differs during walking with various orthoses. In order to improve the performance of these subjects, we need to compare various orthoses according to gait, stability and energy consumption parameters.

Many of the SCI subjects cannot use AFO orthoses. For the specific 'boot' orthosis designed for paraplegic subjects by Kent (1992) a lot of contraindications were considered to select the patients who could use the orthosis. The performance of AFO orthoses for paraplegic subjects is significantly lower than that with other available orthoses (5, 111, 119).

The stability of SCI subjects in standing with traditional HKAFO orthoses is better than with the KAFO orthoses, however the walking speed and stride length of the subjects in walking with the KAFO is greater than those with traditional HKAFO orthoses. Most paraplegic subjects walk with the traditional HKAFO orthosis with swing through gait mechanism however, they can walk with the new designed HKAFOs by a reciprocal gait pattern. The walking speed, stride length and energy cost are higher with swing through gait mechanism than with reciprocal gait (125) however, the force which is applied on the upper limb through the crutch is higher in swing through gait than with reciprocal gait (97, 126, 127).

116

Amongst a variety of the new orthoses designed for paraplegic subjects, the HGO orthosis has the best performance. In comparison with the RGO paraplegic subjects walk with the HGO faster and more comfortable (128). In the HGO orthosis the limbs remains parallel during walking. Moreover, the maximum peak value of the vertical displacement of the pelvis during walking with the HGO is half of that with the RGO and ARGO orthoses (8). The main reason for better performance of the HGO in contrast to other orthoses is its highest lateral rigidity (61).

7.5.2 Comparison between the performance of SCI individuals during ambulation with orthosis and wheelchair

There is no doubt that ambulation with wheelchair has less energy consuming than walking with orthosis. In research carried out by Cerny et al (1980) eleven SCI subjects were selected to walk with KAFO orthoses, with swing through gait pattern, and ambulate with wheelchair. The amount of energy consumption of the subjects used orthosis as the main type of transportation system differed from those who choose wheelchair during walking with orthosis and using wheelchair. Those who walked with orthosis could use wheelchair and the orthoses better than those who used only wheelchair. The mean values of the velocity in using orthosis and wheelchair were 32.4 and 84.9 m/min, respectively. The oxygen uptake in using orthosis was 0.99 ml/kg/m compared to 0.205 ml/kg/m for using wheelchair. The results of this research showed that walking with the orthosis was so demanding because it required a lot of energy and oxygen.

In another research project by Water and Lunsford (1985) the performance of paraplegic subjects with orthoses and wheelchair was compared. A group of normal subjects who walked with a comfortable speed was also included in this study for comparison

117

purpose. The handicapped subjects in this research used different types of orthoses such as, AFO and KAFO orthoses. The results of this research showed that in contrast to ambulation with wheelchair, walking with orthoses is high demanding in terms of energy consumption. There was no significant difference between energy consumption of paraplegic subjects in using wheelchair and normal subjects (walking). So using a wheelchair is highly efficient means of locomotion with average speed, rate of oxygen uptake which is nearly the same as that in normal subjects (5). Table 7.4 shows some results of this research.

The energy expenditure of the SCI individuals during walking with different orthoses and during ambulation with wheelchair was measured by Merati et al (2000). The subjects ambulated with wheelchairs with a velocity between 5.4 and 8.5 km/h however, their speed was 0.59, 0.67, and 0.57 km/h during walking with the Parawalker, RGO and RGO with FES, respectively. The energy consumption of the participants with wheelchairs was less than with orthoses. The results of this research also showed that the energy demand is one of the main problems associated with using orthoses (42).

Parameters	Paraplegics using wheelchair	Paraplegics walking	Normal subjects
Heart rate (beats/min)	123 ±25	138 ±27	100± 14
Speed (m/min)	72 ±17	27 ±17	80 ±11
Oxygen rate (ml/kg/min)	11.5± 3.1	14.5± 4.3	11.9 ±2.3
Oxygen cost (ml/kg/m)	0.16± 0.03	0.74± 0.5	0.15 ±0.02

Table 7.4: Some results of the research done by Waters and Lunsford (2004)

7.6   Problems associated with using different transportation methods

Patients who suffer from SCI have some problems during walking with orthoses or during ambulation with wheelchairs. The main reason for using orthoses is only for therapeutic exercises. However, many of them don't use their orthoses regularly. According to the results of various research studies, SCI individuals use their orthoses especially for standing, but not for performing more purposeful tasks.

The main problem which was stated by paraplegic patients is that walking with orthoses is a demanding task in terms of energy expenditure and the mechanical work required. It is the main reason for avoiding the use of orthoses. Actually the energy consumption in utilization of the orthoses is not high when it used only for standing however, for walking energy expenditure is high and patients have unsustainable fatigue after walking for a short distance.

Another problem that was mentioned by SCI individuals in different research was the cosmesis of the orthosis. The results of the research carried out by Whittle et al (1991) showed that although the HGO orthosis seems to have a better functional performance than the RGO, it was not selected by many patients since it is not as cosmetic as the RGO orthosis.

Donning and doffing of the orthosis is another important problem associated with orthosis usage. Hawana did research by following up 45 SCI patients for 10 years. He found that only 3 out of 45 patients continued using their orthoses. The reason that they mentioned for withdrawing from the use of the orthoses was a considerable of time that they needed to spend in putting on and taking off the orthosis.

The high percentage of the force applied on the upper limb musculature is the other issue that affects the use of orthoses. Depending on the style of walking between 30 % and 55% of BW is applied on the crutch during walking (60, 94, 98, 127). This high value of the force, which is transmitted to the upper limb joints, increases the incidence of some diseases and also shoulders pain.

Another problem which is mentioned regarding unsuitability of the orthoses related to fear of falling, especially during performing hand functions. The stability of the subjects during standing with orthoses must be high enough to allow them to do different hand functions without the need to apply a lot of force on the crutches.

Although the energy expenditure of wheelchair users is nearly the same as that in normal subjects, there are a lot of problems associated with wheelchair use. Bone osteoporosis, joint deformities, problems of musculoskeletal systems are some problems which were mentioned in the literature (30, 33, 35-38, 48, 129). Moreover, they have a lot of problems with architectural features from landscapes. Another problem with wheelchair users is shoulder pain and decreasing the range of motion of the upper limb joints (130). More than 30% of the wheelchair users have shoulder pain and decreased shoulder range of motion (131). Carpal tunnel syndrome is another condition which commonly happens in these patients as a result of repeatable movement with their wrist (130).

CHAPTER 8: SUMMARY

The incidence of the SCI varies between 12.7 and 59 new cases per million each years in the different countries. It is estimated that in the USA between 183,000 and 230,000 are living with SCI, compared to 40,000 in UK. These individuals miss their abilities to stand and walk normally and have to use different transportation methods. The two main types of transportation methods selected by the SCI subjects are using orthoses and wheelchairs.

Although, they can ambulate with wheelchairs using the same energy consumption and walking speed as the normal subjects, they have some problems in using wheelchairs, such as restriction to mobility from architectural features from the landscape and also some health issues arise from using wheelchairs. Some health issues such as bone osteoporosis, joint deformities, shoulder pain, and wrist pain are the main condition associated with wheelchair use.

In contrast to ambulation with wheelchairs walking with orthoses has some benefits for the SCI individuals. Prevention of bone fractures and osteoporosis, improving the functions of the cardiovascular and digestive systems, prevention of joint deformities, and improving the psychological health are some of the benefits of walking with orthoses.

A variety of orthoses have been designed to enable SCI individuals to stand and walk again, which use different mechanisms to stabilize the paralyzed joints and to move them forward during walking. Different sources of powers such as pneumatic and hydraulic pumps, muscular force resulting from electrical stimulation, and electrical motors have been attempted for walking of these individuals. However, the results of different research have shown that the performance of the SCI individuals during walking with the mechanical orthosis is better than other types of orthoses.

Different types of mechanical orthoses are available to help these subjects to stand and walk again however, the two most common ones are the HGO and RGO. The performance of paraplegic subjects while using orthoses was evaluated by gait analysis, energy consumption tests and stability analysis during quiet standing and during performing hand functions. According to the results of different research the performance of SCI individuals during walking with the HGO is better than that of other available orthoses. The main reason is its greatest lateral rigidity of this orthosis in contrast to other available mechanical orthoses.

Although walking with orthoses brings a lot of benefits for these subjects, they prefer to use wheelchairs as a main type of the ambulation method. Many of the SCI individuals withdraw from using their orthoses after they get it. The patients reported some problems such as, walking with orthoses is a demanding task in terms of energy expenditure and the mechanical work required, poor cosmesis of the orthoses, especially the HGO, donning and doffing the orthosis that takes considerable time and sometimes they need assistance, and experience problems related to fear of falling.

In order to improve the performance of SCI subjects during walking and to increase their willingness of them to use orthoses, the aforementioned problems need to be solved. The design of a new orthosis must allow easy donning and doffing of the orthosis by the users, has enough stability during walking and standing, ability of changing the alignment of the orthosis to suit the patient's need, has modular structure, has the maximum lateral rigidity, be cosmetic, decrease the energy consumption during walking, and apply the smallest possible force on the upper limb musculatures during walking.

REFRENCES

1. Stolov WC, Clowers MR. Handbook of severe disability : a text for rehabilitation counselors, other vocational practitioners, and allied health professionals. Washington: U.S. Dept. of Education Rehabilitation Services Administration; 1981.

2. Capaul M, Zollinger H, Satz N, Dietz V, Lehmann D, Schurch B. Analyses of 94 consecutive spinal cord injury patients using ASIA definition and modified Frankel score classification. Paraplegia. 1994;32 (9):583-7.

3. Zampa A, Zacquini S, Rosini C, Bizzarini E, Magrin P, Saccavini M. Relationship between neurological level and functional recovery in spinal cord injury patients after rehabilitation. European Journal of Physical and Rehabilitation Medicine. 2003;39:69-78.

4. Cerny D, Waters R, Hislop H, Perry J. Walking and wheelchair energetics in persons with paraplegia. Physical Therapy. 1980;60:1133-9.

5. Waters RI, Lunsford BR. Energy cost of paraplegic locomotion. Journal of Bone, Joint and Surgery. 1985;67:1245-50.

6. Woolridge C, editor. Spina bifida orthotics program presented at the Workshop on Bracing of Children with Paraplegia from Spina Bifida and Cerebral Palsy1969 2-4 October; National Academy of Sciences, University of Virginia, Charlottesville, VA,.

7. Whittle MW, Cochrane GM, Chase AP, Copping AV, Jefferson RJ, Staples DJ, et al. A comparative trial of two walking systems for paralysed people. Paraplegia. 1991;29:97-102.

8. Jefferson RJ, Whittle MW. Performance of three walking orthoses for the paralysed: a case study using gait analysis. Prosthetics and Orthotics International 1990;14:103-10.

9. Stallard J, Major RE. A review of reciprocal walking systems for paraplegic patients: factors affecting choice and economic justification. Prosthetics and Orthotics International. 1998;22:240-7.

10. Chen HY, Chen SS, Chiu WT, Lee LS, Hung CI, Wang YC, et al. A nationwide epidemiological study of spinal cord injury in geriatric patients in Taiwan. Neuroepidmiology1997;16(5):241-7.

11. Hammell KW. Spinal cord injury rehabilitation. London: Chapman & Hall; 1995.

12. Pickett W, Simpson K, Walker J, Brison RJ. Traumatic spinal cord injury in Ontario, Canada. Journal of Trauma. 2003;55 (6):1070-6.

13. Surkin J, Gilbert BJ, Harkey HL, Sniezek J, Currier M. Spinal cord injury in Mississippi. Findings and evaluation, 1992-1994. Spine. 2000;25 (6):716-21.

14. Sutton NG. Injuries of the spinal cord the management of paraplegia and tetraplegia. London: Butterworths; 1973.

15. Wyndaele M, Wyndaele JJ. Incidence, prevalence and epidemiology of spinal cord injury: what learns a worldwide literature survey? Spinal cord. 2006;44 (9):523-9.

16. NSCISC. Spinal cord injury: facts and figures at a glance. The journal of spinal cord medicine. 2001;24 (3):212-3.

17. O'Connor PJ. Prevalence of spinal cord injury in Australia. Spinal Cord. 2005;43 (1):42-6.

18. Karacan I, Koyuncu H, Pekel O, Sumbuloglu G, Kirnap M, Dursun H, et al. Traumatic spinal cord injuries in Turkey: a nation-wide epidemiological study. Spinal Cord. 2000;38 (11):697-701.

19. Karamehmetoglu S, Unal S, Karacan I, Yilmaz H, Togay HS, Ertekin M, et al. Traumatic spinal cord injuries in Istanbul, Turkey. An epidemiological study. Paraplegia. 1995;33 (8):469-71.

20. O'Connor RJ, Murray PC. Review of spinal cord injuries in Ireland. Spinal Cord. 2006;44:445-8.

21. Maharaj JC. Epidemiology of spinal cord paralysis in Fiji: 1985-1994. Spinal Cord. 1996;34 (9):549-59.

22. Marieb EN. Human anatomy and physiology laboratory manual : fetal pig version. Redwood City, Calif.: Benjamin/Cummings Pub. Co; 1989.

23. Gray H, Carter HV, Pick TP, Howden R. Gray's anatomy. 20th century ed. ed. London: Senate; 1994.

24. Maynard FM, Jr., Bracken MB, Creasey G, Ditunno JF, Jr., Donovan WH, Ducker TB, et al. International Standards for Neurological and Functional Classification of Spinal Cord Injury. American Spinal Injury Association. Spinal Cord. 1997;35:266-74.

25. Lee BY. The Spinal cord injured patient : comprehensive management. Philadelphia, Pa. ; London: Saunders; 1991.

26. Liverman CT. Spinal cord injury : progress, promise, and priorities. Washington, D.C.: National Academies ; Oxford : Oxford Publicity Partnership [distributor]; 2005.

27. Long CI, Lawton EB. Functional significance of spinal cord lesion level. Archives of Physical Medicine and Rehabilitation. 1955;36(4):249-55.

28. Sabo D, Blaich S, Wenz W, Hohmann M, Loew M, Gerner HJ. Osteoporosis in patients with paralysis after spinal cord injury. A cross sectional study in 46 male patients with dual-energy X-ray absorptiometry. Spinal Cord. 2002;40:230-5.

29. Shields RK. Muscular, skeletal, and neural adaptations following spinal cord injury. Journal of Orthopaedic & Sports Physical Therapy. 2002;32:65-74.

30. Rosenstein BD, Greene WB, Herrington RT, Blum AS. Bone density in myelomeningocele: the effects of ambulatory status and other factors. Developmental Medicine and Child Neurology. 1987;29:486-94.

31. Rose Gk, Sankarankutty M, Stallard J. A clinical review of the orthotic treatment of myelomeningocele patients. Journal of Bone Joint Surgery. 1983;65:242-6.

32. Sykes L, Edwards J, Powell ES, Ross ER. The reciprocating gait orthosis: long-term usage patterns. Archives of Physical Medicine and Rehabilitation. 1995;76:779-83.

33. Dunn RB, Walter JS, Lucero Y, Weaver F, Langbein E, Fehr L, et al. Follow-up assessment of standing mobility device users. Assistive Technology 1998;10:84-93.

34. Ogilvie C, Bowker P, Rowley DI. The physiological benefits of paraplegic orthotically aided walking. Paraplegia. 1993;31:111-5.

35. Goemaere S, Van Laere M, De Neve P, Kaufman JM. Bone mineral status in paraplegic patients who do or do not perform standing. Osteoporosis International. 1994;4:138-43.

36. Eng JJ, Levins SM, Townson AF, Mah-Jones D, Bremner J, Huston G. Use of prolonged standing for individuals with spinal cord injuries. Physical Therapy. 2001;81:1392-9.

37. Mazur JM, Shurtleff D, Menelaus M, Colliver J. Orthopaedic management of high-level spina bifida. Early walking compared with early use of a wheelchair. Journal of Bone Joint Surgery. 1989;71:56-61.

38. Rowley DI, Edwards J. Helping the paraplegic to walk. Journal of Bone Joint Surgery. 1987;69:173-4.

39. Carroll N. The orthotic management of the spina bifida child. Clinical Orthopaedics and Related Research. 1974;102:108-14.

40. Kunkel CF, Scremin AM, Eisenberg B, Garcia JF, Roberts S, Martinez S. Effect of "standing" on spasticity, contracture, and osteoporosis in paralyzed males. Archives of Physical Medicine and Rehabilitation. 1993;74:73-8.

41. Middleton JW, Yeo JD, Blanch L, Vare V, Peterson K, Brigden K. Clinical evaluation of a new orthosis, the 'walkabout', for restoration of functional standing and short distance mobility in spinal paralysed individuals. Spinal Cord. 1997;35:574-9.

42. Merati G, Sarchi P, Ferrarin M, Pedotti A, Veicsteinas A. Paraplegic adaptation to assisted-walking: energy expenditure during wheelchair versus orthosis use. Spinal Cord. 2000;38:37-44.

43. Franks CA, Palisano RJ, Darbee JC. The effect of walking with an assistive device and using a wheelchair on school performance in students with myelomeningocele. Physical Therapy. 1991;71:570-7.

44. American Academy of Orthopaedic Surgeons. Atlas of orthotics. 2nd. ed. St. Louis, Mo.: Mosby; 1985. p. 199-237.

45. Redford JB. Orthotics etcetera. 3rd ed. ed. Baltimore: Williams & Wilkins; 1986.

46. Lehmann JF. Biomechanics of ankle-foot orthoses: prescription and design. Archives of Physical Medicine and Rehabilitation. 1979;60 (5):200-7.

47. Rose GK. Orthotics : principles and practice: Heinemann; 1986.

48. Douglas R, Larson PF, D' Ambrosia R, McCall RE. The LSU Reciprocal-Gait Orthosis. Orthopedics. 1983;6:834-9.

49. Lehmann JF, Warren CG, DeLateur BJ. A biomechanical evaluation of knee stability in below knee braces. Archives of Physical Medicine and Rehabilitation. 1970;51 (12):688-95.

50. Kent HO. Vannini-Rizzoli stabilizing orthosis (boot): preliminary report on a new ambulatory aid for spinal cord injury. Archives of Physical Medicine and Rehabilitation. 1992;73:302-7.

51. Solomonow M, Baratta R, Hirokawa S, Rightor N, Walker W, Beaudette P, et al. The RGO Generation II: muscle stimulation powered orthosis as a practical walking system for thoracic paraplegics. Orthopedics. 1989;12:1309-15.

52. Engen T. Lightweight modular orthosis. Prosthetics and Orthotics International. 1989;13:125-9.

53. Lobley S, Rogerson J, Cullen J, Freed M. Orthotic design from the New England Regional Spinal Cord Injury Center. Suggestion from the field. Physical therapy. 1985;65:492-3.

54. Leeder Group I. http://leedergroup.com. 2000.

55. Butler PB, Major RE, Patrick JH. The technique of reciprocal walking using the hip guidance orthosis (hgo) with crutches. Prosthetics and Orthotics International. 1984;8 (1):33-8.

56. Stallard J, Major RE, Poiner R, Farmer IR, Jones N. Engineering design considerations of the ORLAU Parawalker and FES hybrid system. Engineering in Medicine. 1986;15:123-9.

57. Gilbertson MP. Use of the reciprocating brace with polyplanar hip hinge on spina bifida children. Physiotherapy. 1971;57:67-8.

58. Scrutton D. A reciprocating brace with polyplanar hip hinges used on spina bifida children. Physiotherapy. 1971;57:61-6.

59. Stallard J. ORLAU, A brief history- The first 25 years 1975 to 2000: ORLAU 2000 1999.

60. Major RE, Stallard J, Rose GK. The dynamics of walking using the hip guidance orthosis (hgo) with crutches. Prosthetics and Orthotics International. 1981;7:19-22.

61. Stallard J, Major RE. The case for lateral stiffness in walking orthoses for paraplegic patients. Proceedings of the Institution of Mechanical Engineers Part H. 1993;207:1-6.

62. Stallard J, McLeod N, Woollam PJ, Miller K. Reciprocal walking orthosis with composite material body brace: initial development. Proceedings of the Institution of Mechanical Engineers Part H. 2003;217:385-92.

63. Woollam PJ, Dominy J, McCleod N, Stallard J, Major RE. Feasibility study on a composite material construction technique for highly stressed components in reciprocal walking orthoses for paraplegic patients. proceedings of the Institution of Mechanical Engineers Part H. 1999;213:355-60.

64. Ragnarsson KT, Sell GH, McGarrity M, Ofir R. Pneumatic orthosis for paraplegic patients: functional evaluation and prescription considerations. Archives of Physical Medicine and Rehabilitation. 1975;56:479-83.

65. Yongue DA, Douglas R, Roberts JM. The Reciprocation Gait Orthosis in Myelomeningocele. Journal of Pediatrics. 1984;4:304-10.

66. Scivoletto G, Mancini M, Fiorelli E, Morganti B, Molinari M. A prototype of an adjustable advanced reciprocating gait orthosis (ARGO) for spinal cord injury (SCI). Spinal Cord. 2003;41:187-91.

67. Ijzerman MJ, Baardman G, Holweg GGJ, Hermens HJ, Veltink PH, Boom HBK, et al. The influence of frontal alignment in the Advanced Reciprocating Gait Orthosis on energy cost and crutch force requirements during paraplegic gait. Basic and Applied Myology 1997;7:123-30.

68. Davidson HM. The Isocentric Reciprocating Gait Orthosis. APO newsletter. 1994;Sect. 3.

69. David RI, Rolfes RH. Four-bar gait-control linkage. Physical therapy. 1981;61:912-3.

70. Middleton JW, Fisher W, Davis GM, Smith RM. A medial linkage orthosis to assist ambulation after spinal cord injury. Prosthetics and Orthotics International. 1998;22:258-64.

71. Kirtley C, McKay SK. Total design of the walkabout, a new paraplegic walking orthosis. Proceedings, seventh world congress of ISPO; 28th of June to 3th July; Chicago, Illinois USA1992.

72. Genda E, Oota K, Suzuki Y, Koyama K, Kasahara T. A new walking orthosis for paraplegics: hip and ankle linkage system. Prosthetics and Orthotics International. 2004;28:69-74.

73. Kralj AR, Bajd T. Functional electrical stimulation : standing and walking after spinal cord injury. Boca Raton, Fla.: CRC Press; 1989.

74. Goldfarb M, Durfee WK. Design of a controlled-brake orthosis for FES-aided gait. IEEE Transactions on Rehabilitation Engineering 1996;4:13-24.

75. Kagaya H, Shimada Y, Sato K, Sato M, Iizuka K, IObinata G. An electrical knee lock system for functional electrical stimulation. Archives of Physical Medicine and Rehabilitation. 1996;77:870-3.

76. Butler PB, Major RE. ParaWalker: a rational approach to the provision of reciprocal ambulation for paraplegic patients. Physiotherapy. 1987;73:393-7.

77. Sykes L, Ross ER, Powell ES, Edwards J. Objective measurement of use of the reciprocating gait orthosis (RGO) and the electrically augmented RGO in adult patients with spinal cord lesions. Prosthetics and Orthotics International. 1996;20:182-90.

78. Hirokawa S, Solomonow M, Baratta R, D'Ambrosia R. Energy expenditure and fatiguability in paraplegic ambulation using reciprocating gait orthosis and electric stimulation. Disability and Rehabilitation. 1996;18(3):115-22.

79. Ferguson KA, Polando G, Kobetic R, Triolo RJ, Marsolais EB. Walking with a hybrid orthosis system. Spinal Cord. 1999;37:800-4.

80.   Shimada Y, Hatakeyama K, Minato T, Matsunaga T, Sato M, Chida S, et al. Hybrid functional electrical stimulation with medial linkage knee-ankle-foot orthoses in complete paraplegics. The Tohoku Journal of Experimental Medicine. 2006;209:117-23.

81. Gharooni S, Heller B, Tokhi MO. A new hybrid spring brake orthosis for controlling hip and knee flexion in the swing phase. IEEE transactions on neural systems and rehabilitation engineering. 2001;9:106-7.

82. Greene PJ, Granat MH. A knee and ankle flexing hybrid orthosis for paraplegic ambulation. Medical Engineering & Physics. 2003;25:539-65.

83. Dall PM. The function of orthotic hip and knee joints during gait for individuals with thoracic level spinal cord injury [Thesis (Ph.D.)]. Glasgow: University of Strathclyde; 2004.

84. Rose J, Gamble JG, Inman VT. Human walking. 2nd ed / edited by Jessica Rose, James G. Gamble. ed. Baltimore ; London: Williams & Wilkins; 1994.

85. Whittle M. Gait analysis : an introduction. 2nd ed. Oxford ; Boston: Butterworth-Heinemann; 1996.

86. Rose J, Gamble JG. Human walking. 3rd ed. ed. Philadelphia, Pa. ; London: Lippincott Williams & Wilkins; 2006.

87. Murray MP, Drought AB, Kory RC. WALKING PATTERNS OF NORMAL MEN. Journal of Bone and Joint Surgery. 1964;49:335-60.

88. Kadaba MP, Ramakrishnan HK, Wootten ME. Measurement of lower extremity kinematics during level walking. Journal of Orthopaedic Research 1990;8:383-92.

89. Murray MP, Seireg AA, Sepic SB. Normal postural stability and steadiness: quantitative assessment. The Journal of Bone and Joint Surgery. 1975;57:510-6.

90. Winter DA. The biomechanics and motor control of human gait : normal, elderly and pathological. 2nd ed. ed. Waterloo, Ont.: Waterloo Biomechanics; 1991.

91. Nixon V. Spinal cord injury : a guide to functional outcomes in physical therapy management. London: Heinemann; 1985.

92. Somers MF. Spinal cord injury : functional rehabilitation. Norwalk, Conn.: Appleton & Lange; 1991.

93. Somers MF. Spinal cord injury : functional rehabilitation. Norwalk, Conn.: Appleton & Lange; 1992.

94. Melis EH, Torres-Moreno R, Barbeau H, Lemaire ED. Analysis of assisted-gait characteristics in persons with incomplete spinal cord injury. Spinal Cord. 1999;37:430-9.

95. Noreau L, Richards CL, Comeau F, Tardif D. Biomechanical analysis of swing-through gait in paraplegic and non-disabled individuals. Journal of Biomechanics. 1995;28 (6):689-700.

96. Moore P, Stallard J. A clinical review of adult paraplegic patients with complate lesions using the ORLAU Parawalker. Paraplegia. 1991;29:191-6.

97. Slavens BA, Frantz J, Sturm PF, Harris GF. Upper extremity dynamics during Lofstrand crutch-assisted gait in children with myelomeningocele. The Journal of Spinal Cord Medicine. 2007;30(1):165-71.

98. Crosbie WJ, Nicol AC. Biomechanical comparison of two paraplegic gait patterns. Clinical Biomechanics. 1990;5:97-108.

99. Ferrarin M, Pedotti A, Boccardi S. Biomechanical assessment of paraplegic locomotion with hip guidance orthosis (HGO). Clinical Rehabilitation. 1993;7(4):303-8

100. Major RE, Stallard J, Farmer SE. A review of 42 patients of 16 years and over using the ORLAU Parawalker. Prosthetics and Orthotics International. 1997;21:147-52.

101. Baardman G, Ijzerman MJ, Hermens HJ, Veltink PH, Boom HB, Zilvold G. The influence of the reciprocal hip joint link in the Advanced Reciprocating Gait Orthosis on standing performance in paraplegia. Prosthetics and Orthotics International. 1997;21:210-21.

102. Middleton JW, Sinclair PJ, Smith RM, Davis GM. Postural control during stance in paraplegia: effects of medially linked versus unlinked knee-ankle-foot orthoses. Archives of Physical Medicine and Rehabilitation. 1999;80:1558-65.

103. Kaoru A. Comparison of Static Balance, Walking Velocity, and Energy Consumption with Knee-Ankle-Foot Orthosis, Walkabout Orthosis, and Reciprocating Gait Orthosis in Thoracic-Level Paraplegic Patients. Journal of Prosthetics and Orthotics. 2006;18:87-91.

104. Jacobson GP, Newman CW, Kartush JM. Handbook of balance function testing: Mosby Year Book; 1993.

105. O'Connell M, George K, Stock D. Postural sway and balance testing: a comparison of normal and anterior cruciate ligament deficient knees. Gait & Posture. 1998;8:136-42.

106. Raymakers JA, Samson MM, Verhaar HJJ. The assessment of body sway and the choice of the stability parameter(s). Gait & Posture. 2005;21(1):48-58.

107. Lafond DF, Corriveau H, Hebert R, Prince F. Intrasession reliability of center of pressure measures of postural steadiness in healthy elderly people. Archives of Physical Medicine and Rehabilitation. 2004;85:896-901.

108. Goldie PA, Bach TM, Evans OM. Force Platform measures for Evaluation postural control:Reliability and Validity. Archives of Physical Medicine and Rehabilitation. 1989;70:510-7.

109. Kagawa T, Fukuda H, Uno Y. Stability analysis of paraplegic standing while wearing an orthosis. Medical & Biological Engineering & Computing. 2006;44:907-17.

110. Waters RI, Hislop HJ, Perry J, Antonelli D. Energetics: application to the study and management of locomotor disabilities. Energy cost of normal and pathologic gait. The Orthopedic Clinics of North America. 1978;9(2):351-6.

111. Huang CT, Kuhlemeier KV, Moore NB, Fine PR. Energy cost of ambulation in paraplegic patients using Craig-Scott braces. Archives of Physical Medicine and Rehabilitation. 1979;60(12):595-600.

112. Massucci M, Brunetti G, Piperno R, Betti L, Franceschini M. Walking with the advanced reciprocating gait orthosis (ARGO) in thoracic paraplegic patients: energy expenditure and cardiorespiratory performance. Spinal Cord. 1998;36(4):223-7.

113. Yano H, Kaneko S, Nakazawa K, Yamamoto SI, Bettoh A. A new concept of dynamic orthosis for paraplegia: the weight bearing control (WBC) orthosis. Prosthetics and Orthotics International. 1997;21:222-8.

114. Ulkar B, Yavuzer G, Guner R, Ergin S. Energy expenditure of the paraplegic gait: comparison between different walking aids and normal subjects. International Journal of Rehabilitation Research. 2003;26:213-7.

115. Astrand PO, Rodahl K. Textbook of work physiology : physiological bases of exercise. 3rd ed. ed. New York: McGraw Hill; 1986.

116. Bar-On Z, Nene AV. Relationship between heart rate and oxygen uptake in thoracic level paraplegics. Paraplegia. 1990;28:87-95.

117. McGregor J. The objective measurement of physical performance with long term ambulatory physiological surveillance equipment (LAPSE). Proceedings of the third international sysmposium on ambulatory monitoring Academic press. 1979:28-38.

118. Harvey LA, Smith MB, Davis GM, Engel S. Functional outcomes attained by T9-12 paraplegic patients with the walkabout and the isocentric reciprocal gait orthoses. Archives of Physical Medicine and Rehabilitation. 1997;78(7):706-11.

119. Merkel KD, Miller NE, Westbrook PR, Merritt JL. Energy expenditure of paraplegic patients standing and walking with two knee-ankle-foot orthoses. Archives of Physical Medicine and Rehabilitation. 1984;65:121-4.

120. Dall PM, Muller B, Stallard I, Edwards J, Granat MH. The functional use of the reciprocal hip mechanism during gait for paraplegic patients walking in the Louisiana State University reciprocating gait orthosis. Prosthetics and Orthotics International. 1999;23(2):152-62.

121. Kawashima N, Sone Y, Nakazawa K, Akai M, Yano H. Energy expenditure during walking with weight-bearing control (WBC) orthosis in thoracic level of paraplegic patients. Spinal Cord. 2003;41(9):506-10.

122. Ohta Y, Yano H, Suzuki R, Yoshida M, Kawashima N, Nakazawa K. A two-degree-of-freedom motor-powered gait orthosis for spinal cord injury patients. Proceedings of the Institution of Mechanical Engineers. 2007;221:629-39.

123. Baardman G, IJzerman MJ, Hermens HJ, Veltink PH, Boom G, Zilvold G. Knee flexion during the swing phase of orthotic gait: influence on kinematics, kinetics and energy consumption in two paraplegic cases. Saudi Journal of Disability and Rehabilitation. 2002;8:20-32.

124. Baardman G, IJzerman MJ, Hermens HJ, Veltink PH, Boom HBK, Zilvold G. Augmentation of the knee flexion during the swing phase of orthotic gait in paraplegia by means of functional electrical stimulation. Saudi Journal of Disability and Rehabilitation. 2002;8(2):73-81.

125. Cuddeford TJ, Freeling RP, Thomas SS, Aiona MD, Rex D, Sirolli H, et al. Energy consumption in children with myelomeningocele: a comparison between reciprocating gait orthosis and hip-knee-ankle-foot orthosis ambulators. Developmental Medicine and Child Neurology. 1997;39:239-42.

126. Tashman S, Zajac FE, Perkash I. Modeling and simulation of paraplegic ambulation in a reciprocating gait orthosis. Journal of Biomechanical Engineering. 1995;117:300-8.

127. Requejo PS, Wahl DP, Bontrager EL, Newsam CJ, Gronley JK, Mulroy SJ, et al. Upper extremity kinetics during Lofstrand crutch-assisted gait. Medical Engineering & Physics. 2005;27:19-29.

128. Banta JV, Bell KJ, Muik EA, Fezio J. Parawalker: energy cost of walking. European Journal of Pediatric Surgery. 1991;1:7-10.

129. Sabo D, Blaich S, Wenz W, Hohmann M, Loew M, Gerner HJ. Osteoporosis in patients with paralysis after spinal cord injury. A cross sectional study in 46 male

patients with dual-energy X-ray absorptiometry. Archives of Orthopaedic and Trauma Surgery. 2001;121:75-8.

130. Dalyan M, Cardenas DD, Gerard B. Upper extremity pain after spinal cord injury. Spinal Cord. 1999;37:191-5.

131. Subbarao JV, Klopfstein J, Turpin R. Prevalence and impact of wrist and shoulder pain in patients with spinal cord injury. The journal of spinal cord medicine. 1995;18:9-13.

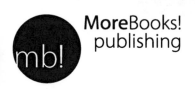
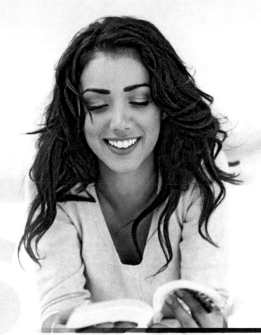

Lightning Source UK Ltd.
Milton Keynes UK
UKOW050459280213

206939UK00002B/255/P